Ayurveda, Nature's Medicine

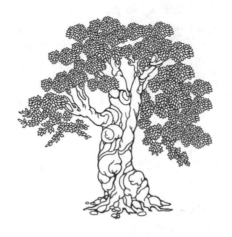

BY DR. DAVID FRAWLEY
&
DR. SUBHASH RANADE

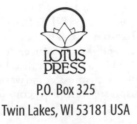

LOTUS
PRESS
P.O. Box 325
Twin Lakes, WI 53181 USA

DISCLAIMER

This guide is not meant to represent definitive guidelines for the treatment of illness or injury. As with any injury or health concern competent professional treatment is recommended.

Cover & Page Design/Layout: Paul Bond, Art & Soul Design

Illustrations: Margo Gal

First Edition, 2000
Reprinted, 2012

Printed in the United States of America

Ayurveda, Nature's Medicine
includes bibliographical references.

ISBN: 978-0-9149-5595-5
Library of Congress Control Number 00-134342

Published by:
Lotus Press
P.O. Box 325
Twin Lakes, WI 53181 USA
800-824-6396 (toll free order phone)
262-889-8561 (office phone)
262-889-2461 (office fax
www.lotuspress.com (website)
lotuspress@lotuspress.com (email)

Table of Contents

Foreword

I have had the good fortune to share the company of and work along side two of Ayurveda's most respected scholars and prolific authors, Dr. David Frawley and Dr. Subhash Ranade.

Dr. David Frawley stands in league with India's most respected historians, yogis and vaidyas. His insights into the knowledge of India's culture, her deep spirituality, and the sacred threads that have woven together thousands of years of mystical tapestry is unparalleled. He has inspired a generation of Westerners to look toward the essence of India's ancient wisdom in the hopes of bringing healing to our own society and our own health care system. A member of the California College of Ayurveda's Board of Advisors, he has been integral in shaping the curriculum of our program and the future of Ayurveda in the West.

Dr. Subhash Ranade is one of India's most prolific ambassadors of Ayurvedic knowledge. His years of clinical practice, time spent teaching, and his many writings have educated physicians and practitioners around the world. I have been moved by his unselfish sharing of India's sacred healing science. Dr. Ranade has worked closely with the California College of Ayurveda to make the knowledge of Ayurveda, long shrouded in mystery, available to Western practitioners.

Here in the West, as the profession of Ayurveda is rapidly growing and formal Ayurvedic education is being made available, there is a need for books that bring to the public a clear and concise understanding of India's indigenous healing system. *Ayurveda, Nature's Medicine* will please both the beginner who is discovering Ayurveda for the first time, and the serious student who desires a clear interpretation of India's ancient knowledge.

Ayurveda has an important role to play in the West. At this time in our history, many people are asking questions about the future direction of our healthcare system. There is less trust and greater dissatisfaction with the existent healthcare system than at any other time in our short history. Paralleling the questioning of "modern medicine" is a burgeoning interest in alternatives that, through natural methods, support the body to reestablish a state of health and well being.

Ayurveda is unique among the many options consumers have today. Its body-mind-spirit approach is not only entirely holistic in its application, but also emphasizes personal empowerment. The great Ayurvedic sage Charaka said, "What the patient knows is more important than what the practitioner knows. The successful Ayurvedic practitioner is not the one who heals the most patients, but the one who teaches his patients to heal themselves."

As a system of self-healing, Ayurveda is unparalleled. Its concepts are profound within their simplicity. Its application, based on common sense, is easy to adapt. Once a person understands even the fundamentals of this great system, their view of the world is changed forever and, with this new perception, reality shifts and healing becomes possible.

Perceiving that the reality we live in is not static but is in fact freely dynamic, capable of change at any time, Ayurveda and its sister science of Yoga explore the nature of that reality and the physical and spiritual principles which shape it. Mastering these principles, a person begins to realize that they are responsible for molding their own reality. Health or disease becomes a conscious choice. On a gross level, it is the direct result of our actions. Most people take action based upon a lack of knowledge of the physical and spiritual laws that govern well-being. Ayurveda teaches us these laws and the actions that go with them so we can establish health within the body, and harmony within the mind, and thus pursue our deeper spiritual goals.

Each one of us has a great potential to live up to. Through our genes and our consciousness, karma sets the stage. What we do once we arrive is up to us. Whether we reach our potential or sabotage ourselves along our journey depends upon the road map that we have in hand. Ayurveda is a map that first helps us to understand who we are and where we have begun. It shows us, too, the end of the journey where we find the ultimate goals of perfect health and enlightenment. Looking at this map, we can see where we are. In front of us are many roads. Some bring us to our goal, others lead us down paths that appear attractive, but which in the end mire us in the web of illusion causing us to forget the inner journey that we are on.

Let Ayurveda help you to remember. In the end, healing is remembering how to be healthy. Enlightenment is remembering how to be whole.

Namaste.

Dr. Marc Halpern
Director, California College of Ayurveda

Preface

Interest in Ayurvedic medicine, India's traditional natural healing system, continues to grow rapidly along with the worldwide return to traditional medicine. In recent years, Ayurveda has taken its place as one of the most important and innovative systems of mind-body healing available. Now many people are interested in learning and becoming practitioners of this profound science of life and establishing Ayurveda as a real medical profession in the West. This trend is bound to continue for decades to come as we enter a new era in which natural healing will supplement, if not begin to surmount, modern biochemical medicine.

This book is designed as an introduction to Ayurvedic medicine, both for interested students, and for informed lay people. It starts out at a basic level but goes thoroughly into its subject. It contains most of the information taught in two-year Ayurveda programs for foreign students in India, but specially oriented to a Western audience. Through it, the reader will gain a broad overview as well as specific views about this ancient science of life and longevity.

The book provides a detailed presentation of all the different branches of Ayurveda and their practical application in daily life. Most importantly, it deals with lifestyle disciplines, including daily, seasonal and yearly practices for optimal health which are the foundation for the Ayurvedic approach to right living.

In particular, we have added a special section on Ayurvedic diets by Dr. Marc Halpern, director of the California College of Ayurveda, who has also most kindly written the foreword.

Dr. Halpern is one of the main pioneers of Ayurvedic education in the West and has worked tirelessly for this cause for several years.

Both of us have been engaged extensively in Ayurvedic teaching programs throughout the world for the last two decades. We hope that this book will be of value both to current and prospective students as well as the general public. Our hope is that it will assist in the proper understanding and application of Ayurveda in the West, and that it will encourage people to take up its practice. May it serve to bring the wisdom of life to its readers!

Dr. David Frawley
Dr. Subhash Ranade

PART ONE

The Ayurvedic Approach to Health

Ayurveda, the Science of Life: Historical and Philosophical Background

He who regards kindness to humanity as the
supreme religion, and treats his patients accordingly,
best succeeds in achieving all the aims of life
and obtains the greatest happiness.

— Sushruta

AYURVEDA AND MEDICINE TODAY

Ayurveda, "the science of life", is the traditional natural medicine of India dating back over five thousand years. It is a science, or way of knowledge about life, its powers and its resources. Yet Ayurveda is not a science artificially imposed upon living beings. Its basis is not found in mere chemistry, or in a mechanistic and materialistic view of the human body. Ayurveda is based upon a deep communion with the spirit of life itself, upon a profound understanding of the movement of the vital force and its manifestations within our entire psychophysical system.

As such, Ayurveda presents a striking alternative to the biochemical model of modern medicine, the limitations of which are becoming increasingly evident through time. We are not simply an accident or a design of chemistry but an expression of a living consciousness that is universal in nature – which is inherently wise and which has the power to balance and transform itself once its nature is understood. Reclaiming that connection with life as a whole is the real basis of healing,

3

not manipulating the life force with drugs, however useful they may be.

Ayurveda is a truly holistic medicine whose great wealth we have just begun to explore in the Western world. It is not merely a kind of antiquated folk medicine as it is sometimes considered to be. It is a science in its own right, with its own rationality and way of experimentation that is extraordinarily intricate and complete. Ayurveda is based upon the observation of living beings and their actual reactions to their environment, not on mere laboratory experiments that seldom address the living being.

Ayurveda classifies all the factors of our lives in an organic and energetic language that reflects the entire living biosphere around us. It shows how our individual constitution and disease tendencies reflect the forces of nature. It shows how foods, herbs, emotions, climates and lifestyles impact the dynamics of our own physiology and psychology that may be different for each person. This enables us to interact with life in an optimal manner both for our own benefit and that of the greater world in a symbiotic manner.

Ayurveda possesses probably the longest clinical experience of any medical system in the world, with a history of Ayurvedic hospitals and colleges going back well over three thousand years. It has carefully examined every sort of disease and life condition and their impact on health and well-being. It contains an intricate and sophisticated system of anatomy and physiology that follows a vitalistic model of the biological humors or doshas that shows us how our life-energies work and how to balance them.

Ayurveda reflects a deep study not only of the body but also the mind and the spirit beyond the mind and body. It reflects an in-depth system of psychology that understands the dynamics of karma and consciousness and how the physical world connects with those more subtle.

For treatment purposes, Ayurveda has created an extensive herbal and mineral industry, offering what is probably the greatest variety of herbal and pharmaceutical preparations available in the world. These include herbal wines, herbal jellies, confections, resins, balsams, various pills and powders, and an extensive system of mineral and alchemical preparations that are unique in the entire world.

Ayurveda possesses a wealth of special clinical procedures, including the use of steam therapy, oil massage, and its own Pancha Karma methods of purification that include everything from enemas to nasal medications. It has special rejuvenation techniques for body and mind that strengthen immunity and retard aging, employing natural methods of diet, herbs, exercise, yoga and meditation.

Perhaps most significantly, Ayurveda uses all these approaches in the context of a greater science of self-care, including an entire methodology of right living for optimum health and the promotion of greater awareness and creativity tailored to the needs of each person. All of this follows a constitutional model that considers the unique nature of the individual as the primary factor in health, not disease as an entity in itself. Ayurveda is a humanistic and person-centered medicine that shows us how to find our own natural health and unfold our deeper energy potentials for the fullness of life, in which drugs and hospitals can become peripheral not primary.

While Western medicine focuses on identifying external pathogens and controlling disease from the outside, Ayurveda concentrates on the living individual and controlling disease through balancing the life-force within the person. As the limitations of antibiotic medicines are now evident today, with weakening immune systems and the return of contagious diseases once thought to be eradicated, such regimens for strengthening our internal energy and immune system are crucial for our health as a species and its survival through future decades. We can no longer simply try to change our environment for health or happiness, as if manipulating the outer will make us feel better on an inner level. We must learn how to develop and improve ourselves and our own internal resources, including not only how we eat and exercise, but also how we breathe and how we think. Ayurveda shows us how to do this and provides us with the knowledge and methods to facilitate the process.

As the traditional medicine of the subcontinent of India, Ayurveda reflects the profound spiritual culture of the region. It is an integral part of Vedic sciences that includes Yoga, Vedanta and Vedic Astrology. It brings us the entire cultural, spiritual and natural wisdom of the Himalayan region with knowledge of how the great yogis and seers cultivated their bodies and minds, and interacted with their natural environment, thus reaching the very source of creation in the cosmic mind.

This ancient and oriental Ayurveda is now spreading world-wide as one of the most important and innovative systems of mind-body medicine available today. As part of the global age, it has left its protective shell in India and is now entering the global arena for the benefit of all peoples. Soon Ayurveda will become an integral part of a new and more humane approach to health care everywhere. In the last ten years, interest in the subject has exploded, with the publishing of many books on Ayurveda and the opening of Ayurvedic centers throughout the Western world, indicating the beginning of a trend that is likely to continue for years to come.

The current crisis in health care, brought about by over-reliance on chemical, mechanical and artificial treatment modalities, now demands the return of the natural, life and soul affirmative systems such as Ayurveda, with their lifestyle regimens for self-healing. Western medicine has become so expensive that it is draining both our personal and national resources. Unless we re-learn the art of self-healing, we will be drowned in drugs, medical testing and chronic diseases that leave us not only unhealthy but also financially insecure. This new move to self-healing is bound to be one of the most important developments in culture and in health care for the coming century.

Ayurveda is ushering in a health care revolution in which lifestyle, diet, exercise and meditation are more important than drugs and surgery, not only for health but also for improving vitality. It is helping us to reclaim our health and our vitality so that we can live the lives that we really want to live and have the creativity and consciousness to make our sojourn on this planet both beautiful and beneficial, not only for ourselves but for all creatures. It is returning medicine to life and to our daily behavior, rather than reducing it to difficult hospital procedures with numerous side effects.

The Meaning and Purpose of Ayurveda

The word Ayurveda has a profound meaning that helps us understand its purpose. "Ayu" refers to all aspects of life from birth to death and all aspects of our nature from body to immortal spirit. It is the continuity and harmony between all that we are and all that we wish to be. "Veda" means knowledge or learning at the deepest level, the wisdom of this conscious universe that we can cognize within ourselves and in our own lives.

Ayurveda is the science by which life in its totality is understood. It describes the diet, medicines, and behaviors that are beneficial or harmful for life and consciousness. It provides a wealth of experiential knowledge and practical healing modalities for all people. Not surprisingly, Ayurveda is called "the mother of all healing" because it cares for all creatures as a mother does for her children. It rejects nothing that is beneficial for life but strives to integrate all valid healing methods in an understanding of how life itself operates.

The sages of ancient India bequeathed Ayurveda to mankind as part of the vast spiritual system of Vedic and yogic knowledge. Seeking out of compassion to alleviate the suffering of all creatures, they looked for all methods of removing pain. They created the system of Yoga to deal with spiritual suffering and Ayurveda to deal with mental and physical suffering. Ayurveda is thus one of the oldest and most comprehensive medical systems in the world, with an unbroken record of clinical experience going back to the dawn of human history.

However, Ayurveda is not only a system of medicine in the conventional sense of a methodology for treating disease. It is a way of life that teaches us how to maintain health and improve both our energy and our awareness – how to live life to our full human and spiritual potential. Ayurveda shows us not only how to eliminate disease but how to promote longevity so that we can realize our goal in life, which is not just gaining material happiness but achieving profound spiritual realization. Ayurveda remains linked to a spiritual view of humanity and contains methods for connecting us to the greater universe that lies both within and around us.

Ayurveda treats the human being as a whole – a combination of body, mind, and immortal soul. It always considers the psychological and spiritual dimension of healing along with the physical in order to address our greater being and manifestation. This makes Ayurveda inherently a truly holistic and integral medical system such as many people are looking for in changing health care circumstances today. As various natural and alternative systems of medicine come to the forefront, and we once more rediscover the power of prayer and meditation, Ayurveda is becoming prominent as a system of medicine that has never forgotten these greater implications of healing. In our examination of Ayurveda, let us first look into the historical and philosophical background of this profound system.

HISORICAL BACKGROUND OF AYURVEDA

Ayurveda and the Vedic Period: 4000 – 2000 BCE

According to the views of India's great sages and yogis, the roots of Ayurveda go back to the very beginning of cosmic creation. The Vedic seers state that Ayurveda originates from Brahma, the creative intelligence behind the universe, from which the entire manifest world comes into being out of unmanifest cosmic laws. The desire to maintain fitness, health, and longevity is a basic instinct born in all creatures and is part of the will of the Creator. We all possess an innate healing power, such as the body demonstrates in its ability to heal itself, and we also have the potential to access and to magnify it.

Ayurveda reflects this medical knowledge inherent in life itself that is coterminous with creation and shows us how to use it in all of its facets. In this respect, Ayurveda sets the pattern for other systems of medicine. It is a tradition with an antiquity comparable to that of life itself. In fact, Ayurveda is said to originate from Prana, the life-force itself, which is the original power behind all creation. Ayurveda is a vehicle for connecting with the cosmic life-force and its unlimited transformative powers.

The *Vedas* are humanity's oldest record of spiritual knowledge, in fact humanity's oldest literature. The latest archaeological information coming out of India over the last two decades shows that the Vedic tradition is over five thousand years old in north India and represents the indigenous culture of the region that has maintained its continuity since the dawn of history. Civilization in India gradually developed from the Mehrgarh village complex of 7000 BCE that shows the beginning of agriculture, the world's first cattle rearing, and other factors that became typical of later Indian civilization. It developed steadily until around 3500 BCE when urban sites and traces of writing first arose.

By the third millennium BCE, ancient India contained the world's largest urban civilization, evidenced by such large cities as Mohenjodaro, Harappa and Dholavira. These sites extended from the Ganges in the east to Afghanistan in the west and from the coast of Iran to the region of Bombay. Originally called the "Harappan" or "Indus" civilization, it is now being renamed the "Sarasvati" or "Indus-Sarasvati" civilization because the great majority of its many sites occur on the banks of the long defunct Sarasvati River. This Harappan or Sarasvati River culture dominated north India until the Sarasvati River dried up, forcing people to move to wetter regions, particularly to the lush Ganges plain to the east. The demise of this river around 1900 BCE owing to geological changes brought this unique culture to an end.

The extensive Vedic literature reflects this Sarasvati culture, lauding the Sarasvati as the greatest river in India, while later classical Indian literature praises the Ganges in a similar way.

Ayurveda arose in the Vedic Sarasvati culture and the earliest Ayurveda is of this era, as reflected in the healing herbs and mantras of the *Vedas*, such as were probably the main medical methods of the Harappan cities.

The *Vedas* state that the Supreme Being who created the Universe out of love and compassion gave the *Vedas* to teach mankind how to live in harmony with universal law (dharma). The *Vedas* teach dharma or right living on all levels from physical health and social relationships to spiritual development. They reflect the power of cosmic creation and hold the keys to cosmogenesis, which includes the power of life and a higher evolution of consciousness beyond the human state to the divine.

The *Vedas* are composed of mantras that embody the very laws and energies of the universe, which are not merely inanimate forces but the powers of consciousness itself. The words of the *Vedas* were carefully memorized according to metrical chants and transmitted from generation to generation over thousands of years. The four *Vedas* – *Rig, Yajur, Sama* and *Atharva* – have come down to us through several thousand years of written and oral transmission.

The *Rig Veda*, the oldest of the four *Vedas*, already contains the main concepts of Ayurveda. Its three greatest Gods or cosmic powers – Indra, Agni, and Soma – relate to the three doshas or biological humors of Ayurveda: Vata (air), Pitta (fire), and Kapha (water). Indra is the deity of the air, atmosphere and Prana or the vital force. Agni is the deity of fire and the sun who consumes or eats all things. Soma is the inner waters of life represented by the moon as being indicative of food and the body.

Soma in the *Rig Veda* also relates to special herbal preparations used to treat the diseases of body and mind and to aid in longevity and rejuvenation. Such Vedic Somas were prepared from the juices of various herbs, particularly those picked from the high mountains, mixed or cooked along with milk, ghee, yogurt, sugar, honey, barley or gold. They were used not only for healing but also for elevating consciousness. While the exact preparation of these Vedic Somas was forgotten over time, Ayurveda preserves similar methods of preparing special herbs and medicines.

The *Yajur Veda* sets forth the Vedic ritual, which among other goals, aims at giving us health and longevity. Those who perform these Vedic practices properly are said to live a happy life of a hundred years or more. Even today Ayurvedic doctors may prescribe such Vedic rituals or yajnas, particularly for dealing with diseases that are difficult to diagnose or to cure. The *Yajur Veda* also introduces the Ayurvedic ideas of the organs and tissues (dhatus) and discusses the five pranas.

The *Sama Veda* sets forth a musical chant that is said to bring health, harmony and well-being to body, mind and soul. Various *Sama Veda* chants (Samans) are credited with gaining special powers over the forces of nature, including the ability to create rain and, on a physical level, to harmonize the forces within the body in order to create longevity and immortality. Even today, Ayurveda stresses the importance of mantra, music and sound therapies for healing at a deep level.

Though all the *Vedas* contain references to Ayurvedic concepts, the *Atharva Veda* contains the most, so much so that Ayurveda is often considered to be an *Upaveda* or branch of *Atharva Veda*. The *Atharva Veda* contains references to specific herbs, the treatment of particular diseases, and other systematic knowledge about Ayurveda. The *Atharva Veda* is the more practical Veda dealing with the needs of daily life and the common people, whereas the other *Vedas* reflect more metaphysical concerns. Its special regard for health and herbs is therefore not surprising.

Ayurveda as an Upaveda or secondary Vedic text is connected with the other Upavedas:

• *Dhanur Veda* – martial arts
• *Sthapatya Veda* – sacred geometry and architecture
• *Gandharva Veda* – music and dance

The other Upavedas are also used in Ayurveda for their healing potentials. Dhanur Veda contains an intricate knowledge of the marmas or sensitive body points on the body and how to make the body strong and fit through exercise. Sthapatya

Veda shows the healing forces inherent in the directions and how to use these in building houses, temples and hospitals. Even today, Ayurvedic hospitals are constructed according to the rules of Sthapatya Veda, also called *Vastu*. Improper Vastu is still regarded as a cause of disease, while proper Vastu helps generate more healing prana in the environment. Gandharva Veda shows how music can heal the body and mind. It remains one of the best methods for treating prana at a deeper level and calming Vata dosha, the biological air humor. Such Vedic music, which is the basis for classical Indian music, is used to balance the elements within us and to harmonize us with temporal changes of day and night and the seasons of the year.

Ayurveda is connected with the *Vedangas* or limbs of the Vedas as well. These six limbs are:

• *Jyotish* – astrology

• *Kalpa* – ritual

• *Shiksha* – pronunciation

• *Vyakarana* – grammar

• *Nirukta* – etymology

• *Chandas* – metrics

Astrology (Jyotish), ritual (Kalpa) and mantra (which are the main concern of the four Vedangas of Shiksha, Vyakarana, Nirukta and Chandas) are important aspects of Ayurveda and reflect these Vedic connections. Of these six Vedangas, Vedic Astrology is perhaps the most significant.

Vedic Astrology is an important aid for the diagnosis and prognosis of disease, showing us when a disease is likely to occur, treatment remedies and prognosis of cure. It is also used in the timing of treatment and in the preparation of medicines, which are stronger if prepared under favorable lunar and planetary influences. Ayurveda and Vedic Astrology are closely intertwined on many levels and work well together as a comprehensive life-therapy. Ayurveda shows us how our life-force works and Astrology delineates the movement of our karma.

Mantra is one of the most important Ayurvedic treatment methods, particularly for the mind and the emotions. Ayurvedic practices are regarded as sacred rituals to put us in harmony with the benefic powers of the cosmos. They are generally sanctified and empowered with special mantras which bring healing forces into the conscious and subconscious mind and the soul.

Later Vedic texts bring in additional Ayurvedic insights. For example, the *Brahmanas* outline the five pranas and the seven tissues in detail. They project a seven-leveled fire altar as the seven aspects of the human being (microcosm) and the seven worlds of the universe (microcosm). The *Upanishads* teach the spiritual and psychological background of Ayurveda and its dedication to self-knowledge and the upliftment of consciousness. The *Mahabharata*, the great epic in which the *Bhagavad Gita* is found, contains specific sections on Ayurveda, explaining the doshas and their effects for both health and disease.

The Ashwini Kumars, the twin horsemen, are the main Vedic deities of Ayurveda, promoting health and rejuvenation on all levels. They are the miracle workers in the *Rig Veda* that heal the sick and raise the dead. These magical twins represent the dual nature of the life-force as expansion and contraction and the need to create balance, which is the essence of all lasting healing. The God Rudra, the Vedic prototype of Shiva, is also important as the original doctor, particularly for curing febrile diseases and for protecting us from injury.

The patron deity of Ayurveda specifically is Dhanvantari, first described in the *Puranas* as a king of Kashi (Benares), who is credited with discovering the immortal secrets of Ayurveda and first establishing the full medical system and propagating it through a school. He is said to be an incarnation of Lord Vishnu, the cosmic power of preservation, who maintains health, harmony and well-being in creation.

FORMATIVE PERIOD OF AYURVEDA:
2000 – 300 BCE

Charaka and Sushruta

After the end of the Sarasvati culture, its knowledge was preserved and gradually reformulated over time. The spiritual and yogic aspect of medicine in the *Vedas* and *Upanishads* was supplemented by observations based upon logic and experimentation. Ayurvedic scholars from subsequent generations explained Ayurveda in a more rational manner, but not forgetting the spiritual roots of the system. The medical material scattered in the *Vedas* was collected, tested for its efficacy and systematically arranged. Such compilations were called *Samhitas*, which literally means collections. Many of these compilations came into being and once existed, but today only three authentic works remain:

* *Charaka Samhita*
* *Sushruta Samhita*
* *Ashtanga Hridaya*

This great trio, or *Brihattrayi* as it is called, has enjoyed much popularity and respect for the last two thousand years. Although these texts underwent modifications and additions in subsequent periods, their core knowledge goes back to remote antiquity. They constitute perhaps the oldest, as well as the longest, medical texts in the world, with a wealth of information on all aspects of life, diet, behavior, herbs, health and disease. They are all written in the Sanskrit language.

 Charaka Samhita (collection of the great teacher Charaka) is the oldest of the three and was probably first devised around 1500 BCE. The book remains the primary textbook of Ayurveda in India today. It describes the fundamental principles of Ayurveda, elaborating the physiological and anatomical structure of the human body, in which regard Ayurveda, emphasizing the living body, has many important insights. Charaka goes into the symptoms and signs of various diseases, including common conditions like diabetes and arthritis that still plague us today. His treatment methods for these diseases using diet and herbs remain sound and helpful.

The book also explains the methodology for examination of patients and prognosis of disease. The preventive aspects of treatment include daily and seasonal regimens, dietetics and social behavior conducive to mental health. The chapter on dietetics in particular is a vast store of information. The section on curative treatments includes detailed descriptions of medicinal plants and their properties, herbal preparations, and therapeutic procedures such as elimination therapy. The chapters on rejuvenation therapy and prevention of the aging process are good sources for modern research work. The *Charaka Samhita* is written in prose as well as in beautiful poetry, comparable to any Sanskrit classic. Charaka represents the Atreya School of physicians, whose approach is mainly herbal.

Sushruta Samhita (the collection of the great teacher Sushruta) represents the Dhanvantari School of surgeons, which emphasizes surgery. In Ayurveda, Sushruta is the father of surgery. A great American society of surgeons today is named after Sushruta in honor of his pioneering work in the field. Sushruta calls surgery the first and foremost specialty of Ayurveda. He describes various surgical procedures including abdominal operations for intestinal obstructions and stones in the bladder, and delineates specialized procedures like plastic surgery. Sushruta was perhaps the first person to advocate knowledge of anatomy through the dissection of the body as essential for a good surgeon.

Sushruta Samhita contains sophisticated descriptions of many surgical instruments. Its classifications of fractures, wounds, abscesses and burns, as well as its procedures for plastic surgery and anal-rectal surgery, have all stood the test of time. Sushruta describes original concepts of pathogenesis of disease. The knowledge of anatomy – bones, joints, nerves, heart, blood vessels, and circulation – is surprising and praiseworthy. The description of the marmas or vital points in the body is comparable to the system of acupuncture points used in traditional Chinese medicine. Sushruta clearly states the importance of both theoretical and practical knowledge and explains ways and means to develop surgical skill.

Later in Indian history, the philosophical emphasis on non-violence, which rejected surgery, got in the way of development of this branch of medicine and it declined. Yet even today, the *Sushruta Samhita* contains a great deal of useful material for research work, and Ayurvedic surgery is still practiced in India, though on a limited scale.

Thousands of medicinal herbs and their products, growing in diverse parts of the country in varied climates, are mentioned in both *Charaka* and *Sushruta Samhitas*. Diseases peculiar to different localities and seasons are found in them as well. *Charaka* and *Sushruta Samhitas* prove that a vast amount of scientific research, patient investigation, and experimentation must have gone on before the conclusions recorded in them were arrived at. This long formative period of Ayurveda may be roughly said to be from 2000 BC to 300 BCE. By this time, great university cities sprang up in India like Takshashila, Nalanda, Ujjain, Mithila and Varanasi (Benares). At this time the eight branches of Ayurveda were developed.

THE EIGHT BRANCHES OF AYURVEDA – ASHTANGA AYURVEDA

Classical Ayurveda as defined in Charaka and Sushruta, like classical Yoga, consists of eight limbs or branches:

1. Internal Medicine (Kayachikitsa)

Internal medicine is the main branch of Ayurveda that treats our entire nature. Ayurveda considers the human being as a whole, comprising body, mind, and soul. Mind and body affect each other and together form the seat of disease. The approach of Ayurveda from the very beginning is psychosomatic. Ayurveda groups all human beings into seven different types of psychophysical constitutions (Prakriti) according to the predominance of the three biological humors (doshas of Vata, Pitta and Kapha). It similarly groups them into seven psychological constitutions according to the predominance of the three mental qualities (gunas of Sattva, Rajas and Tamas).

All these factors are taken into account during the treatment of disease. Diseases are caused by imbalances of the doshas or gunas, which in turn damage various tissues and systems.

Internal medicine mainly deals with diseases that have an internal or organic cause, as apart from injuries or poisons. A number of infectious diseases are described in Ayurveda but great importance is not given to pathogens as their cause. Ayurveda emphasizes internal factors, the condition of the individual behind all diseases, even those appearing to come from the outside. If the soil remains sterile, the seed will not grow. In the same way, if the internal energies are balanced, disease has no field in which to act.

The present book focuses on explaining these factors and their relationship as it is mainly concerned with the internal medicine branch of Ayurveda. This branch of Ayurveda often is regarded as encompassing the rest, which can be seen as aspects of it or additions to it.

2. Surgery (Shalyatantra)

Surgery is not just an invention of modern medicine but was already highly advanced in several ancient cultures, including India, Greece and Egypt. Its low condition in Europe during the Middle Ages was a period of decline, a temporary dark age, and was not indicative of its condition in ancient and Oriental cultures, where it remained more advanced. Ayurveda still contains some forms of surgery but this component of it has been declining. It was taken over more by allopathic medicine in India.

In the field of surgery, modern medicine has made great advances that Ayurveda must acknowledge and admire. But Ayurveda holds that surgery should be integrated with the other aspects of medicine in order to create a truly complete system of medicine. Surgery is not the only method of treatment, nor always the best, but it does have its importance and may have no alternative, particularly in dealing with traumatic injuries or large tumors where it is most appropriate.

3. Shalakya Tantra

This is the Ayurvedic branch of Ophthalmology and Otorhino-laryngology, the branch of medicine dealing with the diseases of the eyes, head and throat. Sushruta described seventy-two eye diseases along with surgical operations for such conditions as cataract and pterygium. Special techniques are described for many diseases of the ear, nose and throat that can be treated locally with various instruments and herbal applications.

4. Pediatrics (Kaumarabhritya)

This branch deals with prenatal and postnatal baby care and with the care of the mother both before conception and during pregnancy. Ayurveda describes special methods for conceiving a child of the desired sex, intelligence, and constitution. Various diseases of children and their treatment come under this branch. According to Ayurveda, the health of children is the key to the health of society. Right diet and exercise for children falls under this branch as preventive methods for diseases likely to occur later on in life.

5. Toxicology (Agadatantra)

This branch deals with the toxins and poisons of the vegetable, mineral and animal kingdoms and how they can adversely affect our health. Most interesting to note is that the concept of the pollution of air and water has been given due consideration. Such pollution is said to be the cause of various epidemics and the collapse of civilizations. Certain poisons, particularly in small doses, also have benefits as medicines.

6. Psychology (Bhutavidya)

Ayurveda is equally concerned with mental diseases and their treatment as it is with physical disorders. Ayurvedic treatment methods include not only physical methods like diet and herbs, but also yogic methods for improving the condition of the mind like pranayama, mantra and meditation. Generally, Ayurvedic doctors prescribe both types of approaches and stress their interrelationship. Bhuta literally means the influence of the past, and shows how previous karmas and mental patterns weigh down the mind and heart. So clearing of negative conditioning from the past is part of this branch of Ayurveda. There is ample material for further research on this branch in the *Vedas, Tantras*, and the Ayurveda *Samhitas*.

7. The Science of Rejuvenation (Rasayana)

Ayurveda addresses all the needs of life, which include how to prolong life and how to renew our vitality after disease or during the aging process. Rejuvenation therapy is used to prevent diseases and for promotion and extension of a healthy life. However, proper detoxification is an essential prerequisite for rejuvenation. A code of right conduct in life also has to be observed as part of the rejuvenation process, including meditation. Details of rejuvenation regimen in terms of diet and herbs have been described in detail in Ayurvedic texts.

8. The Science of Aphrodisiacs (Vajikarana)

Sexual energy is the root of bodily health and disease. This branch of Ayurveda deals with increasing sexual vitality and efficiency necessary for a happy sex life, health and for procreation. For achieving good progeny, the therapy of Rasayana and Vajikarana are closely interrelated. Vajikarana medicines also act as rejuvenatives because the sexual energy can function internally to revitalize our tissues and organs.

These eight branches of Ayurveda overlap and are connected in various ways. So we should not view them as separate but as integral parts of the same approach.

AYURVEDA, BUDDHISM AND AYURVEDA'S CLASSICAL PERIOD: 300 BCE – 1000 AD

The advent of Buddhism in Indian history affected all walks of life. During the period 300 BCE - 600 AD when Buddhism was popular in India, the progress of Ayurveda was well maintained. Various Buddhist authors made valuable contributions to its literature. Most notable was a commentary on *Sushruta* by Nagarjuna, one of the most famous sages and Siddhas in the Mahayana Buddhist tradition who lived in Andhra Pradesh around two thousand years ago. The Medicine Buddha is also figured as one of the great teachers of Buddhist Ayurveda.

Yet the most remarkable thing about this period was that organized efforts were made to make the science as available as possible. Medicinal herbs were planted along the sides of public streets to be used freely by all. Many hospitals were formed. The art of nursing, which was described by Charaka, was widely practiced and systematized.

The knowledge of Ayurveda and of Indian culture spread far beyond the bounds of India. The nations of the then civilized world, including Rome, Greece, Persia and China, were attracted to India and students came from these countries to learn the sciences and arts of the land. The medical systems of Greece and Rome bear signs of the influence of Ayurveda from this period. India was considered the seat of learning for the world philosophers and scholars who visited India for study. Veterinary science was widespread in this period. Nagarjuna laid the foundation of *Rasa Shastra*, the use of alchemical preparations. A number of pharmaceutical preparations of Rasa medicines, special preparations of mercury, sulfur, and other minerals and certain poisonous substances were introduced in treatment.

The medical glory of India was perhaps at its zenith during this era. In the eighth century, Ayurvedic physicians of India were invited to Baghdad in the Middle East for consultation and were put in charge of hospitals there. The culture of India spread across the oceans to the south and east and across the mountains and plateaus to the north. The greater India of that day included Tibet to the north, Indochina and Indonesia to the east, and extended to the west through Afghanistan and into Persia. This greater India was not built by military conquest, nor by invasions or commercial exploitation, but by devoted and humanitarian monks and yogis who carried the sacred knowledge and means of healing, both spiritual and physical, to all who were open to it.

From the second century onward we find an increasing interest in *Rasakriya* or Ayurvedic pharmaceutical chemistry as part of a greater alchemical tradition. During the following six centuries, this study developed into a regular science (Siddha medicine) which was incorporated into Ayurveda. This form of Ayurveda is more popular in the south of India, though aspects of it are used throughout the country.

The next important authority in Ayurveda after Charaka and Sushruta is Vagbhatta of Sindh (the lower Indus valley), who flourished about the sixth century AD. His treatise called *Ashtanga Hridaya* presents a summary of Charaka and Sushruta with gleanings from other Ayurvedic writers and brings the subject up-to-date. He introduced a number of new herbs and made valuable modifications and additions to surgery. The whole book is written in succinct and beautiful poetry, making it easy to memorize. For this reason, it remains a favorite for students learning Ayurveda today. Vagbhatta mentions Buddhist deities and teachers. Tibetan medicine is also based upon commentaries on Vagbhatta.

During this time, the main Ayurvedic texts were translated into Arabic. The Unani or Islamic system of medicine, which the Arabs developed out of the older Greek medicine, was to a great extent founded on Ayurvedic knowledge from India. The Indian Unani system, which grew up under Muslim rule in India, never lost touch with its parental source and even today works with many Ayurvedic herbs and principles.

MEDIEVAL PERIOD AND THE DECLINE OF AYURVEDA: 1000 – 1750 AD

The Muslim invasion of India began in the eighth century and brought about a conquest of most of the country in the thirteenth century. It resulted in a series of devastating wars lasting into the eighteenth century that caused a great decline in the classical culture of India, including Ayurveda. The conquest and its anti-Hindu and anti-Buddhist crusades weakened the older culture and made it difficult to maintain the traditional arts and sciences. Many universities, monasteries and temples, which were repositories of Ayurveda, were destroyed, including Takshashila, Nalanda and Mithila. Faced with this assault, Ayurveda withdrew into the villages and into family centers. Many Ayurvedic teachers retreated to the south of the country or to the Himalayas where there was more safety from the wars.

The medieval period is dominated by the name of Madhava, a great devotee of Vishnu, who in the twelfth century wrote several works embracing almost all branches of Hindu learning from Yoga and religion to Ayurveda. His medical work named *Madhava Nidana* deals exclusively with the diagnosis of diseases. During the Muslim period, up to the eighteenth century, activity in Ayurveda was mainly focused on Rasakriya or alchemical preparations. Chakrapani and Vrinda wrote systematic works on the subject. Narhari Pandita and Madanpal wrote two masterpieces on medicinal herbs, *Raja Nighantu* and *Madanpala Nighantu*. Sharangdhara in the fourteenth century systematized various materia medicas and his is still a most popular and reliable treatise on the subject. *The Sharangdhara Samhita, Madhava Nidana,* and *Bhava Prakasha* are regarded as the *Laghu Traya* or *Junior Triad* of Ayurvedic classics.

The next celebrated writer on Ayurveda is Bhavamishra, the author of *Bhava Prakasha*. This physician lived in the sixteenth century and was considered to be the best scholar of his time. His style is simple and delightful to read. In the time of Bhavamishra, India began to come into contact with the European nations, first the Portuguese, then the French and British.

THE BRITISH ERA: 1750 – 1950

The advent of the British rule in India, which began in the mid-eighteenth century, was a landmark in the further decline of Ayurveda. The British not only denied state patronage to Ayurveda, they took a negative attitude toward the entire system, regarding it as backward or superstitious. The East

India Company closed down all existing schools of Ayurveda in the Indian subcontinent. Yet in spite of suppression and the lack of patronage, Ayurveda remained popular with the masses and still served about eighty percent of the population of the country, passed on mainly through apprenticeship.

This period marked the beginning of Ayurveda's encounter with Western medicine, including not only allopathy but also homeopathy, with which it had a greater affinity.

AYURVEDA IN INDIA TODAY

The national awakening along with the Indian independence movement during the early twentieth century brought about the establishment of national schools and universities and encouraged the revival of Ayurveda. Different state governments in India started regular teaching of Ayurveda and established state boards, faculties and councils of Indian medicine. Modern Ayurveda came to be taught along with allopathic medicine and has sought to explain its traditional methods in modern, scientific terms.

Over fifty universities in India now have faculties of Ayurveda affiliated with over one hundred Ayurvedic colleges. Presently the government of India has initiated a more open policy and allows the founding of more private Ayurvedic institutions. Many new Ayurvedic schools are arising all over the country today. In 1998 the Prime Minister of India, Atal Behari Vajpayee, emphasized the importance of Ayurveda in dealing with the health care needs of the country, particularly of the villages. In the next decade the scope of Ayurvedic education in India is likely to expand greatly.

However, Ayurveda in India today is still given a back seat to allopathy and is often insufficiently funded. For this reason, Ayurvedic schools and hospitals may look inferior to those of modern medicine. It is not the backwardness of Ayurveda that makes them so but the lack of resources to maintain them. Meanwhile, many new Ayurvedic spas have opened in hotels in India, particularly in the south of the country, to provide Ayurveda as a form of lifestyle and health maintenance discipline. These spas are becoming very popular with tourists and foreign Ayurveda students.

GLOBAL AYURVEDA AND THE FUTURE

In the last few decades, Ayurveda has gone global as part of the resurgence of traditional and natural forms of healing. It is now represented by courses and clinics throughout the world with a growing literature in many different languages. Popular Ayurvedic books have appeared in the West by a wide variety of authors. This new interest in Ayurveda is not merely as an ancient form of healing but as a futuristic mind-body medicine that can help us deal with all the stresses and anxieties of our hectic modern lifestyle.

Ayurveda is recognized by WHO (the World Health Organization) as one of the most important medical traditions in the world, necessary for global health. New research on Ayurvedic herbs and treatment methods is occurring in modern medical circles as well. This growing worldwide interest in Ayurveda is helping it to regain its prestige in India, which is still looking to the West for cultural innovations.

The spread of Ayurveda to the West marks an important new era in the resurgence of Ayurveda after a thousand years in which it was under siege. Ayurveda in the twenty-first century looks to re-inherit its glory of ancient times as one of the most important forms of natural medicine practiced in the world. This new global Ayurveda seeks to integrate it into other naturalistic healing modalities, using Ayurveda with its understanding of constitution as an umbrella to bring all forms of healing together. Under Ayurveda's understanding of constitution, all treatment methods have their place and can be recognized for their value. In this way, Ayurveda can employ homeopathy, herbalism, allopathy, acupuncture, chiropractic and other medical modalities.

The global mind is particularly interested in the spiritual

and yogic side of Ayurveda, which is uniquely developed in the system and is notably lacking in Western medical systems. The new global or planetary Ayurveda is also reclaiming its spiritual roots and reconnecting with Yoga, which is already popular worldwide, and with other Vedic sciences like Vedic Astrology. This Ayurveda of the future will take Ayurveda to new heights and make it available for all humanity, not just as a physical medicine but as a complete set of human resources for optimal living and the development of higher consciousness.

PHILOSOPHICAL BACKGROUND OF AYURVEDA

Vedic Systems

Ayurveda is not only a science, but also a philosophy reflecting a deep understanding of the entire universe. All Indian sciences have a basis in philosophy or a view of the meaning of life. Such philosophies are not merely intellectual systems but reflect profound meditative and yogic insight. Ayurveda, which deals with life, observes nature and the universe for its attributes and actions. Ayurveda accepts the Vedic view that the microcosm (individual) and macrocosm (universe) are interrelated and that man is a replica of nature. Hence, Ayurveda is concerned with theories of evolution and the creation of the universe.

The different philosophies of India deal with the process of creation from various points of view. Six systems of philosophy or perception (*Shat Darshana*) called Vedic systems, rely upon the *Vedas* as their authority. There are other Indian philosophies not based upon the Vedas called non-Vedic systems, but even these share a common basis in dharma or cosmic law. Ayurveda mainly derives through the Vedic systems.

Nyaya-Vaisheshika

Nyaya and Vaisheshika are systems of logical philosophy, similar to the classical Western philosophies of Plato and Aristotle. They form the basis of the six systems of Vedic philosophy and their logical and dialectic approaches. They provide some of the prime concepts for Ayurveda. The Nyaya system deals with the means of knowledge, or proofs, and accepts four means of right knowledge:

1. Direct perception via the senses and mind (Pratyaksha)

2. Inference (Anumana)

3. Analogy (Upamana)

4. Testimony or the word spoken by an authority (Shabda)

Ayurveda accepts these four forms of knowledge. Its diagnostic measures are based upon observation and inference. The concepts of the doshas or biological humors reflect the analogy of the elements of air, fire and water. Ayurvedic texts like *Charaka* and *Sushruta Samhitas* are regarded as authoritative testimony on health and disease.

Vaisheshika presents an atomic theory of creation. According to it, earth, water, light (fire), and the principle of motion (air) are based upon elemental particles. The mind also exists as a single atom in every individual. Ayurveda similarly states that the body develops from the union of various elemental particles and that the mind possesses an atomic nature. By changing the composition and relationship between these elemental particles, we can bring health and harmony to body and mind.

According to Vaisheshika, the diversity observable in the universe derives from the transformation of the atoms of earth (gross matter) that results from their contact with heat. Ayurveda accepts this theory and states that all the transformations in the body, both creative and destructive, occur owing to the existence of the fire principle (Agni) in the body. If this heat principle is normal, health is maintained and if it is abnormal, disease results. Death occurs when Agni ceases to function in the body.

According to Vaisheshika, substances, qualities and actions increase similar conditions in the body. This is the simple principle of *like increases like*. Antagonistic substances, qualities and actions decrease these same factors. This is the principle of *treatment through opposites* – that conditions are generally balanced or cured by an application of opposite qualities. For maintaining health and curing disease, one has to understand these similarities and contraries. The Ayurvedic principle of treatment is to use either similar or antagonistic means according to the requirements of the condition. This is another principal brought from Vaisheshika.

Ayurvedic pharmaceutical theory is based upon the Vaisheshika description of substance, quality and action (dravya, guna, and karma). Substances (dravya) create actions (karma) according to their qualities (guna). For example, hot substances like steam produce hot actions like sweating according to their qualities, which is to increase heat. Ayurveda describes twenty qualities to explain the action of foods and herbs. All substances are applied according to the principles of similarity and contrariety.

Samkhya and Yoga

Samkhya and Yoga form the second pair of Vedic philosophies and have a deeper and more spiritual orientation. Yoga is represented by the Raja Yoga system of Patanjali in the *Yoga Sutras* which is regarded as the main text of the Yoga school. Patanjali codified the older yoga tradition into two hundred brief aphorisms. The original founder of the Yoga system was the legendary sage Hiranyagarbha.

Samkhya is the cosmological and philosophical view behind Yoga. Its founder is the legendary ancient sage Kapila, who existed before Buddha and Krishna. Its main text is the *Samkhya Karika* of Ishvara Krishna (a figure different from the Krishna of the *Bhagavad Gita*), who lived in the early centuries AD. Just as Patanjali compiled the older Yoga tradition in the form of his *Yoga Sutras*, so Ishvara Krishna compiled the older Samkhya tradition in the *Samkhya Karika*. *Samkhya Karika*, like *Yoga Sutras*, is a key text not only for students of Samkhya and Yoga but also for those of Ayurveda.

Though it uses important principles from Nyaya-Vaisheshika, Samkhya and Yoga provide the background philosophy and main principles for Ayurveda. The Samkhya theory of creation does not stop at the level of five elements like that of Vaisheshika, but outlines the working of the mind and senses. It ultimately posits two eternal principles of Primal Nature or Prakriti and the inner Self or Purusha, pure consciousness.

Samkhya teaches that Prakriti is composed of the three gunas, or qualities, of Sattva, Rajas, and Tamas - the principles of harmony, disturbance and inertia. These gunas exist behind all substances in the universe which are ultimately forms of experience for consciousness. Everything is a manifestation of Sattva, Rajas or Tamas.

Samkhya describes the different levels of knowledge through which we can understand both ourselves and the world around us. Five categories of knowledge exist at the level of the five sense organs relative to the five different sensory impressions of sound, touch, sight, taste and smell. These reflect the five elements of ether, air, fire, water and earth.

Three categories of knowledge exist at the level of the mind – pleasurable, neutral, or painful. Samkhya explains these according to the three gunas: Sattva brings lasting happiness, Rajas causes pain in the long run (though it may bring short-term pleasure), and Tamas creates dullness or lack of feeling.

The process of knowing occurs at the level of the intellect (buddhi), which determines right and wrong, true and false, good and bad. Yet the intellect is merely an instrument and is not itself the origin of knowledge. There must be another principle responsible for knowing and it must be ever-knowing. Samkhya calls this principle the *Purusha* or pure consciousness and looks to it as the basis of our self-identity. Our sense of self does not derive from any external object or even from our body but is inherent, spontaneous and self-existent, deriving from consciousness itself.

The Purusha is the ultimate subjective principle of consciousness, just as Prakriti is the ultimate objective principle of materiality. These two, Prakriti and Purusha, are the ultimate, causeless, omnipresent, and all pervasive causes of the universe. When they combine, creation starts and when they get separated, creation comes to an end. The ending of creation according to Samkhya is the merging of creation back into its origin or the effect back into its cause (Prakriti).

The soul in living beings reflects the Purusha, while the material vestures including body, mind and intellect derive from Prakriti. The aim of Samkhya is to provide detachment and liberation to the Purusha, by helping us understand both Purusha and Prakriti and her manifestations. The permanent detached state of the soul is the absolute state of joy or ananda that is everlasting. Yoga provides the methods to purify the mind in order to help bring this about.

Ayurveda accepts the absolute detachment of the soul and describes the highest goal of treatment as the state of liberation in which the soul is no longer bound to the space-time creation and regains its immortal nature. Yet Ayurveda also considers the state of Prakriti or our mind-body condition as the foundation for pursuing liberation, which requires physical vitality and mental insight in order to realize. Ayurveda does not advise neglect of the body, but stresses the need to maintain it and infuse it with vigor in order to achieve both the worldly and spiritual goals of life. At the same time, Ayurveda recommends self-restraint to cultivate detachment and to make efforts for Self-realization.

Ayurveda considers the Purusha (soul) associated with Prakriti (the body or material nature) as the real individual for the practical purposes of treatment. This is the soul in its state of bondage as apart from the transcendent Purusha beyond all sorrow. It is the soul associated with mind, prana and body. In this way, Ayurveda addresses the needs of all levels of people, not just those seeking liberation, who are usually few in this material world.

From these two basic principles of Prakriti and Purusha, Samkhya outlines the main principles of existence, shown in the following table:

Purusha – Pure Consciousness

1. Nature – Prakriti (Composed of three gunas)		
2. Mahat or Buddhi – Intelligence or Intellect		
3. Ahamkara – Ego or I-sense		
Sattvic Ahamkara Vaikritika (Diversified)	Rajasic Ahamkara Taijasa (Radiant)	Tamasic Ahamkara Bhutadi (Origin of Elements)
4. Manas (Mind) 5-9. Five Sense Organs of ears, skin, eyes, tongue and nose 10-14. Five Motor Organs of speech, hands, feet, emission and reproduction	Interrelationship Through Prana	15-19. Five Tanmatras or sensory impres-sions of sound, touch, sight, taste and smell 20-24. Five Elements of earth, water, fire, air and ether

Ego or Ahamkara is the root of all the diversity that we experience both subjectively and objectively. So too, the way to harmony is to transcend ego to our deeper soul and intelligence that is not limited or disturbed by the ego's involvements.

Ayurveda uses this scheme of the sense organs, motor organs, tanmatras, elements and gunas, accepting the Samkhya system of the tattvas or cosmic principles. Ayurveda, one could say, is the Samkhya vision projected into the biological sphere.

In addition, Samkhya teaches the law of transformation (Parinamavada). Prakriti, as a composition of the three gunas, is always in a state of flux. Due to the endless combinations of these three basic qualities, changes occur at every moment. Ayurveda accepts this law of transformation and explains it as the reason for creation and destruction, occurring both in the body and in the external world. It aims at helping us understand the nature (Prakriti) of both body and mind so that we can use their natural transformations to further our goals in life.

The three gunas of Samkhya are very important in Ayurvedic thought and treatment, particularly for the mind. Increase in Sattva, the quality of purity, gives right knowledge to the intellect, provides courage and determination to avoid harmful things and gives an alert memory. Ayurveda recommends various methods to increase Sattva by the regulation of diet and behavior. On the other hand, an increase in either Rajas or Tamas, the qualities of agitation and dullness in the mind, is responsible for wrong decisions, fearfulness and loss of memory. Rajas and Tamas are the mental doshas or toxins that cause psychological disease, which in turn contributes to physical disease.

The Yoga system aids Ayurveda by providing it specific methods for increasing Sattva, decreasing Rajas and Tamas, and balancing the mind. To achieve this, Yoga provides a regimen called yama and niyama, various ethical and lifestyle principles like non-violence, truthfulness, cleanliness and contentment. Yogic methods of asana, pranayama and meditation are included in Ayurveda both for lifestyle practices and for the treatment of disease, particularly of a psychological nature, and can be very important healing methods. Indeed, Yoga therapy, using the methods of Yoga to treat disease, is traditionally part of Ayurveda, which itself can be called "yogic medicine".

Ayurveda uses other yogic approaches including devotion (Bhakti), knowledge (Jnana) and Tantric modalities, adapting the whole range of yogic approaches from ritual and mantras to formless meditation. These are also important parts of its rejuvenation therapy and its treatment of the subtle body. Note the chapter on "Yoga and Ayurveda."

Vedanta and Mimamsa

The third pair of Vedic systems is *Mimamsa* and *Vedanta* (also called *Purva Mimamsa* and *Uttara Mimamsa*). Mimamsa explains the ritualistic interpretation of the *Vedas* and prescribes various rituals, mainly fire offerings, for obtaining happiness in this world and in the after life, including rituals to cure disease and promote longevity. Vedanta deals with the ultimate liberation of the soul and its union with God, which occurs through meditation.

These two philosophies have also contributed to Ayurveda. Mimamsa states that every soul or Purusha is everlasting and travels through the great cycle of birth and death. One experiences pain or pleasure according to the deeds or karmas performed in this or previous lives. The incurability of certain diseases is explained in Ayurveda by this law of karma. Not all diseases are amenable to physical or even to psychological treatment. Some diseases occur owing to karma and must be experienced, or can only be alleviated by spiritual or religious purification methods, like charity, prayer and meditation.

The Ayurvedic view of the inherent freedom of the Soul (Atman) from all bonds of sorrow and the ultimate union of the individual soul with the universal soul is taken from Vedanta. Ayurveda, like Vedanta, is based upon the principle of self-knowledge and aims at self-realization, the knowledge of the One or Divine Self in all beings. Ayurveda directs us back to our True Nature beyond time and space as the ultimate source of all healing, peace and happiness. This is the basis of the Yoga of knowledge (Jnana Yoga), such as taught by the modern teacher Bhagavan Sri Ramana Maharshi.

Theistic Vedantic systems also exist and are very important to the Yoga of devotion (Bhakti Yoga), worshipping the Creator in diverse forms as Vishnu (including Rama and Krishna), Shiva, Devi (the Goddess) and other forms like Ganesh and Hanuman. These various forms reflect the different temperaments of human beings and different spiritual paths, covering the full range of relationships with the Divine as father, mother, beloved, friend or master. This allows each individual to worship the Divine in whatever form and manner that they choose.

Ayurveda recognizes the role of the Creator, and that worship and prayer have great healing powers for both body and mind. It also recognizes that different forms of the Divine are more appropriate for certain individual constitutions than for others, and that finding the right form of the Divine to worship greatly improves our health and vitality. These views it derives from theistic Vedantic systems.

Non-Vedic Philosophies and Ayurveda

While Ayurveda is based primarily on Vedic philosophies, it was also used from the perspective of Buddhist, Jain and other non-Vedic philosophies, from which it has borrowed certain points. These philosophies share many common themes with the Vedic systems like the principle of Dharma (natural law), the belief in karma and rebirth, and the practice of Yoga and meditation. They similarly emphasize non-violence and natural healing. They differ mainly in philosophical ideas as to the nature of ultimate reality.

Both Buddhist and Jain systems are non-theistic and do not posit a Creator. They see karma alone as the cause of living beings. Vedic systems contain theistic systems that posit a Creator (Ishvara), but also non-theistic systems as well (for example, many forms of Samkhya are non-theistic). Jainism recognizes a Purusha (higher Self) but not a Supreme Being or pure existence (Brahman) as do most Vedantic systems, and sees the liberation of the individual Purusha as the highest goal. In this regard, Jainism resembles Samkhya. Buddhism does not posit an Atman or Purusha (higher Self) and regards the non-Self (Anatman) as the highest reality. However, it does recognize a higher awareness or Buddha mind that in many respects resembles the Vedic Purusha that is similarly a state of pure seeing and pure awareness.

Jain thinkers state the law of uncertainty, or all probabilities (syadvada), holding that any number of points of view are always possible on any subject. From the standpoint of diagnosis and treatment, Ayurveda accepts this law of probabilities. One cannot definitely know all such factors and so one's approach should always be flexible. There is no ultimate or final diagnosis or treatment but just various angles of approach, each with its own particular value and its limitations.

If one approach does not work, one should try another.

Jainism emphasizes non-violence or ahimsa as the supreme principle. Ayurveda strives to create a healing approach that is free of violence, cruelty and harm to other creatures and to the environment. That is why it emphasizes vegetarian diet and herbal medicine. Most Buddhist and Vedic systems emphasize non-violence as well.

The Buddha teaches that creation is a momentary affair. Each thing gets destroyed in the following moment. Ayurveda uses this law as a part of treatment. A disease gets destroyed of its own accord and health gets reestablished when the causative factors that produce the disease, like wrong diet, are eliminated. Ayurvedic treatment seeks to remove the cause of disease so that health will return automatically.

Buddhism teaches emptiness or Shunyata as the ultimate truth. Ayurveda recognizes that emptiness, space and silence have great healing potentials for the body as well as for the mind. Buddhism also lauds compassion. Ayurveda is based upon compassion, the desire to see an end of suffering for all creatures, as part of its motivation for practice.

Since all the important Indian philosophies have contributed to the development of Ayurveda, a study of their principles is helpful for all students of Ayurveda. Ayurveda has a place for the knowledge found in all the great philosophies of the world because its aim is the maximum integration of human knowledge toward the maximum fulfillment of life. It has room for all views that promote healing, balance, harmony, understanding and peace.

Ayurveda says that just as different individuals require different diets, so too they require different philosophies and spiritual paths. What is a good spiritual path for one person may not be good for another, just as the diet and behavior for one type may not work for another. In this way, different names and forms of God and the Goddess, or theistic and non-theistic approaches can all be harmonized as each has its value. Reflecting the great abundance and diversity of nature, Ayurveda recommends a free and pluralistic approach to truth so that each person can find what is appropriate for their own unique nature and potentials on all levels from health to self-realization. Ayurveda, like the beauty of life, embraces all points of view in a higher harmony of creation and transformation.

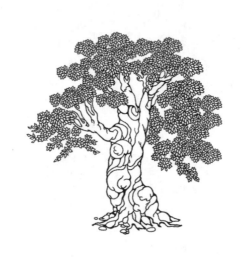

2

The Enduring Principles of Ayurveda

There is no end to learning Ayurveda. You should carefully and constantly devote yourself to its study. Increase your skill by learning from others without jealousy. The wise regard the whole world as their teacher, while the ignorant consider it to be their enemy.

—*Charaka*

Ayurveda is a science of positive health and fulfillment in life. It aims at providing us the optimal energy and intelligence to live long and happily and to contribute to the welfare of the world. It helps us understand the effects of all our actions from eating and sleeping, to work and study, prayer and meditation. The aim of Ayurveda is threefold:

• To achieve positive health for the individual
• To aid in the upliftment of society
• To facilitate ultimate liberation of the spirit

Ayurveda offers daily and seasonal health regimens for achieving optimal health. These show us how to adjust our behavior to best benefit from our individual nature and from the unique circumstances of our lives. This additional energy should be used not only for improving our own life expression, but also to help others less fortunate than ourselves and to engage in spiritual practices to raise the consciousness in the world. In this way, Ayurveda helps us develop energy for the benefit of all creatures.

This Ayurvedic approach is based upon extending our basic urge to preserve our life. From birth we possess the instinct to protect the body from pain and harm. Similarly, our mind possesses an instinct to avoid suffering and conflict. To remain continuously healthy and achieve liberation involves eradicating all the factors that bring about sorrow. Ayurveda identifies these factors and provides practical methods to remove them. It teaches us how to master our character and the outer circumstances of our lives.

Ayurveda bases itself upon an understanding of universal substances, particularly the five great elements of earth, water, fire, air and ether, which do not change their properties. The Moon and water act as cooling agents, while the Sun and fire function to increase heat. The properties of such forces are demonstrated naturally as a matter of common experience. Proof by laboratory techniques is not required. For example, we do not need an experiment to prove that fire burns; its burning quality is evident in all that it does. We must learn to observe all the energies at work in our lives in a similar way.

The drugs employed in modern medicine have been changing rapidly since their inception, while the basic nature of the human body continues to remain the same. The medicine of one generation therefore becomes ineffective or even harmful for the next. The antibiotics that help one generation become the bane of another. When the drugs used for a short period of time cease to be helpful, it indicates that there is something fundamentally wrong with our entire approach to healing, that we have not penetrated to the enduring principles behind life. Contrary to this variability in modern medicine, the principles and methods of Ayurveda have remained constant through time. This is because Ayurveda proceeds from an understanding of the unchanging laws of the universe, rather than merely from following human invention.

Ayurveda recognizes a common origin for the universe and for humanity. The human being is a miniature replica of the greater world and contains the same forces of creation and destruction. The universe is a single organism with a single consciousness and is itself a living being.

For the creation of the universe, two types of substances are required – material and nonmaterial. Material substances create the outer form of things, while nonmaterial factors provide their inner qualities. Material substances, like the five elements, are responsible for the measurable aspect of things, while nonmaterial substances or ideas impart their meaning. Both substances are present in each person.

The Three Gunas or Primary Qualities of Nature

Nature consists of three primary qualities, called gunas in Sanskrit, as introduced in the discussion of Samkhya and Yoga in the previous chapter.

1. Sattva	Consciousness or intelligence
2. Rajas	Motion or action
3. Tamas	Inertia which resists them

These three inner qualities exist behind all material forms in Nature. Their contribution is essential for the creation of anything in the universe. Underlying idea (Sattva), motivating energy (Rajas), and sustaining inertia (Tamas) are the three factors behind the existence of any substance. These three primary qualities, being common to all forms, do not possess a specific form of their own and are known only by their effects. They are called "nonmaterial substances" because they have no particular form but still are a kind of substance or principle of objectivity.

The three gunas manifest in human beings in our temperament, constitution and behavior, which reflect either intelligence (Sattva), agitation (Rajas) or inertia (Tamas). The gunas determine the quality of our lives and whether we are growing in consciousness (Sattva), expanding in ego (Rajas), or simply stagnating in ignorance (Tamas). They are the primary essences behind all that we do, through which we can understand the direction and motivation of our lives. According to Samkhya philosophy, the gunas underlie all aspects of Nature (Prakriti) starting with cosmic intelligence (Mahat).

THE FIVE GREAT ELEMENTS

The five great elements (Pancha Mahabhutas) of ether, air, fire, water, and earth form the basic material constituents of both the universe and the human being. These elements refer to the etheric, gaseous, radiant, fluid, and solid states of matter and their respective principles of space, movement, light, cohesion, and density. They are not merely elements in the chemical sense but different densities of matter. The elements themselves are much subtler than their visible counterparts on Earth. They are the prime substances from which different objects are made, unlike the gunas that are the qualities or ideas according to which they are made.

The elements, we could say, provide the clay from which a pot is made, while the gunas are responsible for making it beautiful or ugly. While the elements provide the quantitative aspect of things, like their size and density, the gunas are responsible for their qualitative meaning. According to the Samkhya system, the elements evolve from the ego (Ahamkara), which is the force of differentiation latent in creation.

Each of these prime elements possesses a characteristic property through which we can apprehend it through the senses. The knowable property of ether is sound; that of air is touch; that of fire is sight; that of water is taste; and that of earth is smell. We grasp these properties through the corresponding five sense organs of the ear, skin, eye, tongue, and nose. Each element similarly possesses a secondary property that can be felt through the skin. These are non-resistance (ether), vibration (air), change of temperature (fire), fluidity (water), and shape (earth). The skin can feel the effects of all five elements indirectly.

The Five Elements

Elements	Sanskrit Name	Primary Property	Secondary Property	Characteristic
Ether	Akasha	Sound	Non-resistance	Subtlety
Air	Vayu	Touch	Vibration	Movement
Fire	Tejas	Appearance	Heat and Color	Transformation
Water	Apas	Taste	Fluidity	Liquefaction
Earth	Prithivi	Smell	Solidity	Density

TRIDOSHA THEORY:
The Three Biological Humors

Ayurveda explains all bodily functions relative to corresponding movements in the outer universe. The three main forces in the external world are the Sun, Moon and Wind that govern all processes in nature. The Sun is the energy of transformation represented by fire. It relates to Pitta or the biological fire humor in the human being. The Moon is the agency of cooling represented by the combination of earth and water. It relates to Kapha, the biological water humor within us. The Wind is the principle of movement or propulsion represented by the combination of air and ether. It relates to Vata, the biological air humor. The Sun causes things to grow through its heat and light. The Moon nurtures things through its watery and emotional influence. The Wind stimulates things by its movement and fluctuations.

All activities in the universe occur according to the three basic functions of creation, preservation, and destruction. These are the actions of three main Hindu Gods of *Brahma*, *Vishnu* and *Shiva* - the Creator, Preserver and Destroyer of the universe. These three functions also relate to the three bio-

Vata Body Type	Pitta Body Type	Kapha Body Type

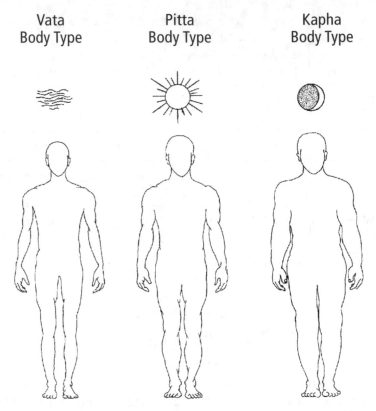

logical humors or doshas. Vata, the energetic humor, controls destruction. We can observe this destructive action of Vata or Wind in earthquakes, hurricanes, cyclones and tornadoes. Pitta, the thermogenic humor, builds up the body after the transformation of food through the process of digestion. This is akin to fire constructing landmass through volcanic action. Kapha, the cohesive humor, is responsible for maintaining the creation, which is why the body consists mainly of water.

Relationship of the Five Elements to the Three Energy Principles in the Universe

Wind - Vata Dosha	Air and Ether, Movement & Space	Principle of Propulsion
Sun - Pitta Dosha	Fire, Energy	Principle of Conversion and Transformation
Moon - Kapha Dosha	Earth and Water, Density & Cohesion	Principle of Preservation

Relationship of Elements, Gunas and Doshas

Ether	Sattva
VATA	Sattva + Rajas
Air	Rajas
Fire	Sattva + Rajas
PITTA	Sattva + Rajas
Water	Sattva + Tamas
KAPHA	Sattva + Tamas
Earth	Tamas

From Ether as pure sattva the other four elements evolve, with Earth as pure tamas. Air is the principle of motion (rajas). Fire has both sattva (illumination) and rajas (heat and passion). Water has sattva (transparency and receptivity) and tamas (inertia). All events observable in the universe are caused by one of these three energies:

- Vata – Agency of propulsion
- Pitta – Agency of transformation
- Kapha – Agency of cohesion

The energy of propulsion causes changes in position, like clouds in the sky that follow the direction in which the wind blows. In the body, functions like respiration, heartbeat, and the expulsion of waste products are manifestations of change in position. In the mind, this function is motivation, through which mental activities take place. These follow the movement of Vata dosha or the air-humor.

While the energy inside the body is termed Vata, which means "wind", Vata should not be simply equated with wind as a physical force. Vata as wind is an analogy. Vata is any propulsive force and the principle of movement generally on the level of the life-force (Prana). The seat of this dosha is the lower part of the large intestine or rectum. The function manifested in this organ, the drying of waste matter by removing the liquid portion, resembles the desiccating effect of the wind.

When a substance comes in contact with the heat of the Sun, it changes temperature, form, appearance or taste. In the human body, the same type of thermogenic energy transforms the food consumed into tissues and waste products. It is responsible for the complexion of the skin and the temperature of the body. This force is called Pitta, meaning "that which cooks or transforms things". Sweat, which is increased by heat, and blood, which is red in color, having properties common to fire, are the main seats of Pitta. Pitta also governs perception, which is the illuminating power of the mind.

The effects of the two energies of Vata and Pitta are inhibited by a third force, the agency of cold and cohesion, which in Nature functions as the rainfall. This force is responsible for growth and sustenance. Hence, it is named Kapha, meaning "that which gets activated by water". The plasma, watery secretions, muscular tissues, bony structures, and the nervous and reproductive systems are the chief sites of this dosha, which constitutes most of the substance of the body. It also imparts feeling to the mind, which is our ability to hold things on an emotional level.

Doshas, Tissues and Waste-materials

Ayurveda classifies all body constituents into three main categories:

1. doshas

2. tissues – dhatus

3. waste-materials - malas

The doshas are the energizing forces, the tissues (dhatus) provide substance, and the waste-materials are the excess that is eliminated.

Waste products (malas) are substances continually being removed from the body. Their physical appearance varies from gaseous, liquid, and semi-solid to solid form. The gross waste products are urine, feces and sweat. Subtle waste products are exudations eliminated from the linings of the eyes, nose, mouth, ears, and reproductive organs. The many minute waste products formed in the body during tissue formation are included among subtle waste-materials. Health is maintained when all waste products are properly eliminated. When they accumulate in excess, they damage the tissues and produce various diseases.

Tissues (dhatus) are bodily constituents that do not get eliminated from the body (with the exception of the reproductive tissue). They are maintained within the limit of the skin from the outside and the mucus membranes from the inside (of the gastrointestinal tract, lungs, bladder, joints, and cerebral linings). As bodily strength grows, these tissues continue to develop. They are seven in number, with characteristics and functions as follows:

The Seven Tissues or Dhatus

NAME	CHARACTER	FUNCTION
PLASMA - Rasa Dhatu	Circulating nutrient; fluid	Nutrition
BLOOD - Rakta Dhatu	Hemoglobin portion of blood	Oxygenation of the blood
MUSCLE - Mamsa Dhatu	Muscle Tissue	Movement
FAT - Meda Dhatu	Adipose tissue	Lubrication

The Seven Tissues or Dhatus

NAME	CHARACTER	FUNCTION
BONE - Asthi Dhatu	Supporting and accommodating bony structures	Support
NERVE AND MARROW - Majja Dhatu	Tissue within the bones: Nerve and bone marrow	To promote understanding
REPRODUCTIVE TISSUE - Shukra Dhatu	Reproductive secretions	Reproduction

The tissues provide support and strength to the body. The body cannot afford to eliminate them like the waste-materials. If they cross over the limit of the skin or the internal linings of the mucus membranes, the disease condition becomes serious because essential substances are lost.

The doshas play a dual role between waste-materials and tissues and have characteristics of both. The doshas do not continue developing like the tissues, nor are they completely eliminated from the body like the waste-materials. In normal amounts, they strengthen the body like the tissues, while in excess amounts they become toxins like un-eliminated waste-materials.

Vata dosha has no physical form, but is perceived by the various movements that it sets in motion or by the effects that it causes (like dryness). Pitta and Kapha both possess a fluid character. Pitta consists of lighter and warmer fluids, like bile and blood. Kapha comprises the heavier and cooler fluids, like mucus, fat and plasma that congeal into denser forms.

FORMATION OF THE DOSHAS

Formation of Vata

The action of swallowing enables us to take in food from the external world. This movement is ongoing and depends upon previously digested food, which creates the need for more food to sustain the processes already set in motion by previous eating. This results in a continual process of eating, digesting and elimination. A direct relationship exists between energy and food absorption. The more energy that we require to function, the greater the need for the proper food to sustain it, for example, needing to eat more when we are doing hard physical work.

Vata dosha is described as the by-product of the digestion of food, which includes the energy produced by digestion as well as the waste gases of the digestive process. Anna Mala, the ejectable portion from food, equals Vata dosha or the portion of Vata that is produced. This absorbed energy is then utilized by the body for essential movements like breathing, heartbeat, digestion, and excretion of waste products, which are the main actions of Vata. These movements cannot be measured or weighed. Thus, Vata is perceived by the totality of its functions. However, if Vata is produced in excess it becomes a negative factor, drying or disturbing the various tissues and organs.

Formation of Pitta and Kapha

The secretions that appear in the upper part of the gastrointestinal tract disappear in its lower portion during the process of digestion. Saliva and mucus secretions (Kapha) and other digestive fluids, including various enzymes and acids (Pitta), occur in the mouth, stomach and small intestine. These are reabsorbed in the small and large intestines along with the digested food. In this way, Kapha and Pitta arise and disappear as part of the digestive process.

Kapha dosha is the ejectable product from the plasma or the nutrient body fluid or plasma (Rasa Dhatu) from which most bodily secretions arise. *Rasa Mala, the excess product of the plasma equals Kapha dosha*. Such Kapha loses certain characteristics of the plasma and aids in lubrication, tissue formation and elimination. When this Kapha leaves the circulating channels as a nutrient fluid, it forms various tissues according to the needs of the body. It may change into muscle tissue, or provide its lubricating material for adipose tissue, or help in the formation of bones, nerves, and reproductive fluids. The channeled nutrient fluid of Kapha aids in the cohesion of various tissues. Yet it can also undergo pathogenic changes, becoming mucus that clogs the chest or head.

Pitta dosha is the product of the breakdown of the blood (Rakta Dhatu). *Rakta Mala, the excess product of the blood equals Pitta dosha.* Pitta appears as colored secretions in the middle portion of the gastrointestinal tract and is responsible for the main digestive function. The blood is different from other tissues in that it does not combine with other constituents in the body. Pitta, however, which is a breakdown product of hemoglobin, is different from the blood in that it aids in various conversions; in the eye for vision, in the skin for complexion, and in the liver for formation of various tissues. Yet in excess, Pitta becomes a toxin that causes various sorts of inflammation or fever.

PROPERTIES OF THE DOSHAS

The doshas are known by their properties:

> *Vata dosha is dry, cool, rough, depleting, propulsive, subtle and astringent in taste.*

When the living body, which is basically watery in nature, comes into contact with such Vata qualities, it becomes weakened or depleted. However, even though these qualities can be harmful to existing tissues in the body, they are essential for certain body functions. For example, if the subtleness of a tissue is completely eliminated, movement in it is impaired leading to congestion and failure of essential bodily functions.

> *Pitta dosha is slightly oily in character, has a sharp odor, with secretory and vasodialating properties, and is penetrating, hot, pungent and sour in taste.*

In the process of digestion, Pitta becomes an easily flowing fluid. All colors except white, dusky or violet, denote Pitta, which like fire, possesses color. Pitta strengthens the body by digesting food but can weaken it by creating excess heat that burns up the tissues or causes bleeding.

> *Kapha dosha is oily, cool, smooth, soft, heavy, nourishing, slimy, compact in arrangement, white in color, and sweet or salty by taste.*

Kapha is the substantial or material component of the three doshas and easily accumulates in various liquid and semi-solid forms. It shapes and sustains the body but in excess causes stagnation and build up of excess tissues, mucus, fat and water.

FUNCTIONS OF THE DOSHAS

Functions of Vata Dosha

As the principle of propulsion, Vata carries out diverse functions in the body and mind. It controls cell arrangement and division, the formation of different tissue layers, and the differentiation of organs and systems. It conducts impulses from the sense organs to the brain and from the brain to the motor organs. Vata controls the expulsion of feces, urine, sweat, menstrual fluid, semen, and the fetus. It regulates respiratory, cardiac and gastrointestinal movements, as well as all higher functions in the brain and spinal cord. Vata governs the movement of the mind and its transmission of information and provides the energy to perform all mental activities of thought and perception.

Functions of Pitta Dosha

Pitta is responsible for the formation of tissues, waste products, and energy from the food, water, and air that we take in from the outside world. It controls metabolic activities and governs all secretions that occur in the gastrointestinal tract and the enzymes and hormones that flow from ductless glands into the blood stream. Pitta regulates body temperature, hunger, thirst, fear, anxiety, anger, and sexual desire, which are all stimulated by heat. Psychologically, Pitta is responsible for courage and will power, and assimilation of knowledge from the outside world (mental digestion).

Functions of Kapha Dosha

Kapha increases the deposits in the cell mass and is essential for the inter-linking of cells, tissues, and organs. It is responsible for the growth and sustenance of the body. Kapha prevents the destruction of tissues from wear and tear due to friction and movement by Vata, maintaining the flexibility, strength and immunity of the body. Capacities for reproduction, happiness, emotional calm, and the correct retention of knowledge depend upon the proper functioning of Kapha, which has a stabilizing and nurturing action on both body and mind.

The proper interrelationship of the three doshas is necessary for health. They are mutually interactive, increasing and decreasing in a proportional manner relative to each other. Generally, Vata and Kapha are opposite each other as light and heavy, function and substance, while Pitta mediates between the two as the power of converting one into the other. Although these forces are in a constant state of flux owing to the impact of internal and external factors, their equilibrium is usually maintained. When this equilibrium gets disturbed, the disease process starts. According to Ayurveda, all diseases are caused by disturbed doshas. Even traumatic diseases that are not initially the result of doshic imbalances soon become accompanied by them, usually first by aggravating Vata which is the most sensitive of the doshas.

SUBTYPES OF THE DOSHAS

Vata, Pitta and Kapha have five subtypes or five subdoshas each, according to their specialized functions.

Five Types of Vata Dosha

The five types or subdoshas of Vata, also called *Vayus*, are: *Prana, Udana, Vyana, Samana* and *Apana*. All these forms are responsible for various movements.

Prana – Udana

These two forms of Vata, having opposite movements, oper-
ate together. Prana Vayu moves from the outside to the inside.
Prana is responsible for receiving air, water, food, and impressions from the outside world. Whenever a sound, touch, taste,
or smell is attended with concentration, it has an effect on
respiration (Prana). Prana Vayu moves downward from the
head into the body. In the process, it brings in various external
forms of nourishment and energy from food and breath to
impressions.

Udana Vayu moves from the inside to the outside, mainly
through exhalation and speech but also through various forms
of exertion. Food and water received by the stomach, rendered
fine during digestion, are eliminated to some degree through
expiration. Speech, which occurs through exhaling air through
the vocal cords, is due to Udana. Memory, which is the bringing out of the knowledge that has been previously received by
Prana, is also a function of Udana. Thus, Prana is responsible for
intake and Udana for output. Udana governs will, enthusiasm
and motivation. Udana moves upward from the center of the
body up to the head and is centered in the throat.

Vyana – Samana

These two types of Vata also have opposite movements. Vyana
Vayu is responsible for propulsion from the center to the periphery of the body. The movement of the heart in pushing
nutritive substances to the periphery is a function of Vyana.
It governs circulation to the limbs and the flow of blood and
sweat. Vyana carries efferent impulses from the sense organs
to the brain. Vyana pervades the entire body from its center in
the heart. Physical exercise and extension of the limbs occurs
mainly through Vyana.

Samana Vayu, on the other hand, is the propulsive force
from the periphery to the center. Afferent impulses in the
nerves, bringing the fluid pushed out by Vyana back to the
center and promoting the process of digestion, are functions of
Samana. Thus, the action of Samana is the central pull action
opposite the outward push of Vyana. We could say that Samana

is centripetal force, while Vyana is centrifugal force. Samana is centered in the navel and is responsible for the churning action in the intestines through which we digest our food.

Apana

In contrast to the above two pairs, Apana controls all downward discharges of urine, feces, flatus, menstrual fluid, semen, and the fetus. All these are controlled for a particular period of time before being discharged from the body. The overall control of these substances for a particular period is beneficial for building or maintaining the tissues. Since this control is beneficial to the other types of Vata, it is said that Apana controls all the different forms of Vata. Apana also sustains the immune function that rests upon proper elimination. Apana moves downward from the navel. It is often regarded as opposite Prana as eating is opposite elimination, or as opposite Udana (upward movement) as downward movement.

Five Types of Pitta Dosha

The five types or subdoshas of Pitta are: *Pachaka, Ranjaka, Alochaka, Sadhaka* and *Bhrajaka*. All these are responsible for some type of digestion, which process occurs on various levels throughout the body and mind.

Pachaka Pitta

Pachaka Pitta is responsible for the primary conversion process in the body, the digestion of food. It makes up the stomach acids, bile salts and other digestive juices. Because of its hot and penetrating quality, it disintegrates and digests food in the gastrointestinal tract.

Ranjaka Pitta

Ranjaka Pitta aids in the secondary digestion of food for the formation of tissues. The formation of blood (Rakta) and other tissues in the liver is the chief function of Ranjaka Pitta, which colors the blood and other secretions.

Alochaka Pitta

Alochaka Pitta is responsible for the assimilation and conversion of visual stimuli that take place when an object is sensed by the eyes. Sensations of sound, touch, taste, and smell also require the proper digestion. The factor responsible for this digestion of impressions is Alochaka Pitta.

Sadhaka Pitta

Sadhaka Pitta is located in the brain and works through the nervous system. After sensing any object, its recognition is dependent upon a specific sequence of conversions in the brain cells governed by Sadhaka Pitta. The capacity to appreciate art is another function of it. Sadhaka Pitta works to digest ideas and experiences in the brain, particularly in the cerebrum.

Bhrajaka Pitta

Bhrajaka Pitta maintains the temperature and complexion of the skin, and helps in the absorption of sunlight, oils and ointments through the skin. Its condition is reflected by the lustre of the skin.

Five Types of Kapha Dosha

The five types or subdoshas of Kapha are: *Avalambaka, Kledaka, Bodhaka, Tarpaka* and *Sleshaka*. All these protect various organs from wear and tear due to the dryness of Vata and the hot and penetrating effects of Pitta. Similarly, they help maintain the cohesion and inter-linking of tissues.

Avalambaka Kapha

Avalambaka Kapha protects the lungs, heart, and upper portion of the intestines. Due to repeated contraction and relaxation of these organs, they are subject to friction and wear. But the fine, slimy and smooth secretions inside these organs protect them and preserve their integrity.

Kledaka Kapha

Kledaka Kapha protects the upper and middle abdomen from hot, irritant or cold food as well as from the secretions of Pachaka Pitta. It exists in the form of alkaline digestive secretions.

Bodhaka Kapha

Bodhaka Kapha protects the mouth from pungent, hot, cold or irritating food and drinks. It also helps us taste food properly. Potentially harmful substances are initially rejected by this taste screen. It also helps the other sense organs in the head that require their fluid lining for protection.

Sleshaka Kapha

Sleshaka Kapha lubricates all the bony ends of the joints and prevents their friction during movement of the limbs. It reduces wear and tear during physical movement. When it is reduced joint pain and arthritis occur.

Tarpaka Kapha

Tarpaka Kapha provides various nutrients to the brain cells and gives lubrication and protection to the brain and spinal cord. It cushions the nerves from stress and harm. It allows us to feel emotional ease and contentment.

PRANA, TEJAS AND OJAS

Prana, Tejas and Ojas are the subtle or master forms of Vata, Pitta and Kapha that govern positive health and vitality. They are refined forms of the subdoshas of Prana Vayu, Sadhaka Pitta, and Tarpaka Kapha and have similar functions governing the mind, vitality and nervous system. Prana is the positive or health-giving aspect of Vata. Tejas is the positive or health-giving aspect of Pitta. Ojas is the positive or health-giving aspect of Kapha.

Ojas itself is the essence of all the tissues as the essence of the reproductive tissue. It holds our primal energy reserve and our congenital strength and sustains our immune function. Ojas, which is a very subtle oily substance, when heated creates Tejas which is the fire of courage, willpower and motivation. Tejas in turn generates energy or Prana, which here means the master Prana governing the functions not only of the body but also of the mind. This higher Prana is our creative force that allows for long-term healing and for rejuvenation, as well as for spiritual growth. Prana, Tejas and Ojas are part of a deeper

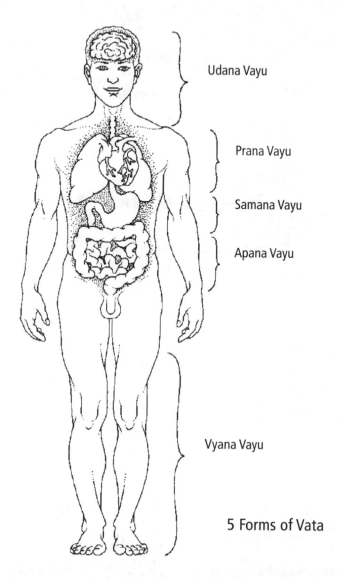

Udana Vayu

Prana Vayu

Samana Vayu

Apana Vayu

Vyana Vayu

5 Forms of Vata

level of healing that requires working with subtle energy.

DIGESTION OF FOOD

Agni - The Digestive Fire

Agni refers to the universal principle of transformation in all its forms, which we most commonly experience in the outer

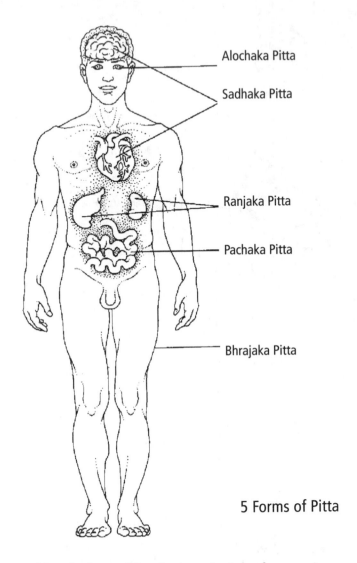

Alochaka Pitta

Sadhaka Pitta

Ranjaka Pitta

Pachaka Pitta

Bhrajaka Pitta

5 Forms of Pitta

world in the form of fire. Such a principle of conversion appears throughout the universe in the various changes of substances observed in biochemical, chemical and nuclear processes. It serves to transform the gross into the subtle, in which process energy is released and new forms are created.

Agni, the digestive fire, represents this power of transformation in the physical body. Agni serves to convert food into various bodily constituents. This conversion takes place

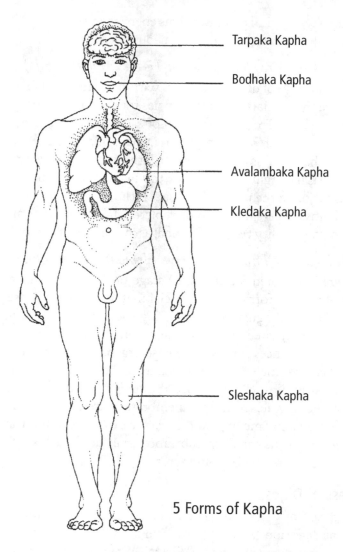

Tarpaka Kapha

Bodhaka Kapha

Avalambaka Kapha

Kledaka Kapha

Sleshaka Kapha

5 Forms of Kapha

by three types of Agni working at three different levels in the body, resulting in thirteen types of Agni:

1. Jatharagni; 2 – 8. Dhatvagnis; 9 – 13. Bhutagnis.

1. The Digestive Fire (Jatharagni)

The digestive fire is the agency responsible for digesting food in the small intestine. It is also called "Kayagni," or the bodily fire, because it is the main source of heat in the body. It supports all other physiological processes. This energy converts the food ingested into a uniform or homogeneous mass.

2-8. Digestive Fires for the Seven Tissues (Dhatvagnis)

The second stage of digestion occurs within the tissues. Dhatvagnis are the special digestive agencies for the various bodily tissues (Dhatus). For the formation of each tissue, a separate Dhatvagni is required, making seven Dhatvagnis for the seven tissues. Dhatvagni is dependent on Jatharagni. If the activity of the Dhatvagni is too low or too high, it results in the malformation of the particular tissue. If the tissue Agni is too high, the tissue gets burnt up or depleted. If it is too low, an excess of low quality tissue is formed, as in the case of tumors.

9 –13. Digestive Fires for the Five Elements (Bhutagnis)

Bhutagni is required for the third stage of digestion, which brings about the formation of special materials for the sense organs. Five Bhutagnis exist for taking the five element portions of the digested food mass and converting them into nutritive substances for the five sense organs. Some of these specialized materials are the rods and cones responsible for photosensitivity in the eye, special liquids around the taste buds on the tongue, the mucus membrane material inside the nose that aids in smelling, and special cartilage forming the architecture of the ear. Such substances specific to each sense organ are prepared by the Bhutagnis.

Process of Digestion

The process of digestion has two components, the primary phase of digestion (Avasthapaka), which is its main portion, and the post-digestive effect (Vipaka), which is its ultimate result. The primary phase of digestion (Avasthapaka) is divided into three stages, according to the prevalence of tastes (rasas) operative during them.

1. Sweet Stage – Stomach – Kapha

The sweet stage of digestion (Madhura Avasthapaka) is the stage of liquefaction. During this stage, Kledaka Kapha secretions occur in the mouth and stomach and the disintegration of the food gradually takes place. Due to the heavy secretionary action of Kledaka Kapha, there is a reduction of activity in the body after eating.

2. Sour Stage – Small Intestine – Pitta

The sour digestive stage (Amla Avasthapaka) is the stage of acidification. Secretions of Pachaka Pitta, digestive juices and enzymes, which occur mainly in the small intestine, break down the food further, marking the central portion of the digestive process. Pachaka Pitta causes a sensation of thirst and perspiration through its creation of heat.

3. Pungent Stage – Large Intestine – Vata

The pungent digestive stage (Katu Avasthapaka) is the stage of alkalization of food. About four and a half hours after eating, the food passes into the lower part of the gastrointestinal tract, the large intestine, and peristaltic movements are diminished. The water is absorbed from the stool, which takes shape for its elimination. During this stage, there arises a desire to move about in contrast to the inactivity of the first phase of digestion. This stage involves a transient predominance of Vata.

The post-digestive effect (Vipaka) is similarly described in three categories. It can be sweet (Madhura Vipaka), sour (Amla Vipaka), or pungent (Katu Vipaka), depending upon the qualities of the particular food eaten.

If a sweet post-digestive effect is formed, then the body receives nutrition of all types and excretory products have the proper lubrication to be easily discharged. Sour post-digestive effect indicates that the body will be only moderately nourished but waste products will still be eliminated smoothly. Pungent post-digestive effect means that the body neither receives proper nutrition nor easily eliminates waste products owing to the dryness characteristic of this phase. Thus, the post-digestive effect denotes the ultimate result of digestion.

The doshas reflect the rhythms of time that govern all the movements of life. They show how the forces of nature discharge their effects according to different time periods and various processes of transformation.

In the cycle of the day, Kapha is dominant in the morning and evening, the formative periods when energy is developing. Pitta predominates at noon and midnight, the peak or transformational hours. Vata is highest at sunrise and sunset, the transitional points of the day.

Seasonally, Kapha is highest in late winter and early spring, the seasons of cold, dampness and early growth. Pitta is highest in the late spring and summer, the season of heat and maturation. Vata is highest in the fall and early winter, the seasons of cold, wind and dryness when energy declines.

In the digestive process, Kapha is highest immediately after eating, when Kapha secretions like saliva form in the mouth and stomach. Symptoms like nausea or belching right after food intake indicate high Kapha. Pitta is highest two or three hours after eating, when Pitta secretions form like bile form in the small intestine, at which time it may be experienced as hyperacidity or heartburn. Vata is highest at the end of the digestive process, four to six hours later, when the food moves into the large intestine, evidenced by symptoms like gas or constipation.

The doshas are constantly changing and interacting, so that even a Vata person will have Kapha or Pitta periods, just as a Kapha person or a Pitta person will have times in which the other doshas will predominate within them. For this reason, we should not take constitution rigidly and should remain aware of secondary doshic fluctuations within each type.

Movement of the Doshas through the Cycle of Time

	KAPHA	PITTA	VATA
DAY	7 am - 11 am	11 am - 3 pm	3 pm - 7 pm
NIGHT	7 pm - 11 pm	11 pm - 3 am	3 am - 7 am
YEAR	Feb. 7 – Jun. 7	Jun. 7 - Oct. 7	Oct. 7 - Feb. 7
DIGESTION	1st 1 ½ hour	2nd 1 ½ hour	3rd 1 ½ hour

3

Individual Constitution: Prakriti

1. AYURVEDIC (BIOLOGICAL OR DOSHIC) CONSTITUTION

Have you ever looked at yourself and then looked at the people around you and seen how much you resemble certain individuals but are very different from others? It is clear that there are tremendous variations among human beings both physically and psychologically and these must be considered for both health and happiness. Ayurvedic treatment is based upon understanding the individual constitution involved. It regards the condition of the living individual, the actual human being, as the most important factor in both health and disease.

Ayurveda does not regard disease as existing in itself but occurring as a complication of constitutional imbalances rooted in the nature and behavior of the individual. According to its view, disease is more a product of internal malfunctions than a result of external pathogens. The state of our internal energies determines our predisposition to external disease factors that are always present in the environment to some degree.

The predominance of the doshas at the time of conception decides the mind-body type of an individual, called *Prakriti* in Sanskrit. Once set, this proportion generally remains permanent for one's lifetime. However, constitution is influenced by environmental factors: Class, family traits, place of birth, time, age, and individual action, which can modify the birth constitution. The birth constitution depends upon the following:

• Condition of sperm and ovum at the time of conception
• Condition inside the uterus
• Food and lifestyle of mother during pregnancy
• Nature of the elements comprising the fetus.

Seven types of constitutions can be formed based upon the permutations and combinations of the three doshas. These types are classified by their predominance. A purely single dosha constitution is seldom found and although a balanced constitution is very good, this type is also rare.

Seven Constitutional Types

Vata	Kapha	Vata-Kapha
Pitta	Vata-Pitta	Pitta-Kapha
Balanced constitution (Sama Prakriti, VPK)		

Vata constitution is usually more difficult in terms of health and longevity because of Vata's inherent instability and weaker vitality. Pitta generally falls in between, with the fire of Pitta aiding digestion but also aggravating febrile and infectious diseases. Kapha constitution is usually superior in health, giving good endurance and stamina, provided Kapha people avoid obesity which weakens their inherent strength and makes them prey to many diseases.

Of the dual constitutions, Pitta-Kapha type is generally best for health, combining the heat of Pitta with the stamina of Kapha. Vata-Kapha type is more difficult, being very susceptible to cold, which quality both Vata and Kapha share. Vata-Pitta is usually the most difficult type because it lacks the Kapha or tissue support to maintain health. A balanced constitution (Sama Prakriti), in which all three doshas are in equal proportion, is better.

However, best of all is to know one's constitution and manage it properly. Whatever one's constitution, one must strive to keep it in balance and if one makes the proper adjustments, optimal health can be maintained. Generally, Vata types are more willing and able to make changes which compensates for their generally lower vitality. Pitta types are moderate in making changes and will do so once convinced of the need. Kapha types are the slowest to make adjustments to their health problems, which can compromise their stronger constitution and turn it from an asset into a liability.

VATA Constitution

Vata type individuals usually have tall or thin bodily frames with less bodily strength and poorer endurance. Their body weight is low and their tissues, like blood and muscle, are not well developed. Their digestion and metabolism is variable and changeable, making it difficult for them to form sturdy and stable tissues. Similarly, their resistance to disease and to the external elements like heat and cold is less, making them easily disturbed by weather changes.

A typical Vata temperament is nervous and sensitive and so Vata types often cannot perform their tasks steadily and continuously. They may fail in achieving their goals or become sidetracked in what they do. However, they are blessed with much enthusiasm and creativity and if they can direct these consistently they can achieve a lot in life. Such individuals require a job with less strenuous physical activity, where constant attention is not required, and which is not located in a cold or dry environment. They do well at creative and communication work with a variety of tasks to perform.

If they are forced to undertake hard work, they are likely to get diseases of the nerves and bones, and to suffer from constipation, along with loss of weight. They need to be treated with care and consideration because their minds and bodies are fragile.

PITTA Constitution

Pitta types have average builds and bodily frames, with good circulation and warm extremities. They possess quick and strong digestive systems that enable them to eat and digest a great variety of foods without unduly putting on weight. They require constant food and drink that is cool and moist in nature to keep them from overheating. Though they are able to convert food into good quality tissue, because the total conversion rate in the body is very fast, they can burn themselves out and feel depleted.

Pitta types have skin that is soft, oily, and smooth. They tend to become bald or prematurely gray at an early age. Their eyes are sharp and penetrating and their features are often angular. They have average strength and capacity for work, although they are hot tempered and quickly become irritable if things do not go their way.

Pittas have good comprehension and are very intelligent and perceptive. They usually possess good knowledge in their chosen subjects, are natural leaders, and often possess wealth and status in society. They require a job in a cool atmosphere, with some important activity and intelligent work aligned with their motivation.

KAPHA Constitution

Kapha individuals possess hefty, robust and thick body frames, with a stout musculature. Their flesh, bones, hair and teeth are well developed. They naturally have good strength, strong immunity and vitality, are generally healthy and have a longer life span. The total digestive and metabolic rate in these individuals is slow and they require less food or drink than other types. For this reason, they put on weight more quickly than other types even if they do not eat a lot. They have smooth and deep voices and are often good looking. Their nature is calm and quiet but they get easily attached both to people and possessions.

Kapha types can carry out work that is heavy or strenuous but may need to be stimulated into doing it. They are good at maintaining public relations and bringing people together and like to care for others. They are generally successful in the long run and accumulate wealth and possessions for themselves and their family. However, they should not work in cold and damp environments, which causes their energy to stagnate. They are prone to become obese which results in joint diseases, diabetes or heart problems.

Physical Structure and the Five Elements

The predominance of the five elements in a person creates the physical structure and the relative proportion of the limbs and tissues. This is determined by those elements present at the time of conception and generally follows the predominant dosha. Kapha is watery in terms of elemental structure, Pitta is fiery, and Vata is airy. The description of these doshic types applies to their respective elemental types. Earth constitution is generally categorized under Kapha and ether constitution under Vata, but they also have their particular characteristics as described below.

EARTH CONSTITUTIONS have a body that is bulky, heavy, square and thick. Their bones are usually large and there may be a significant amount of body hair. They possess strong endurance and are good workers but can lack leadership skills, motivation or enthusiasm.

ETHER CONSTITUTIONS have lightness and looseness in the body, with clear senses and open external orifices. They have a lot of insight and sensitivity but can be impractical or ungrounded in what they do. While their minds are well developed, physically they can lack stamina and substance. They have good mental, artistic or spiritual inclinations.

2. MENTAL (GUNIC) CONSTITUTION

The predominance of sattva, rajas and tamas in the mind decides the mental nature and a person's level of spiritual development. This is based upon the gunas prevalent at birth, which reflects the karma or past life actions of the soul. As a mental factor, the gunic condition is more easily changed by life activity and learning. It is not as constant as the doshic constitution. It also fluctuates relative to daily, seasonal changes and social interaction and so must be observed over time. We all possess sattva, rajas and tamas to various degrees, even if the qualities of one guna dominate in our nature.

Sattvic Constitution

When Sattva or the quality of harmony prevails in a person, one is intelligent, sensitive and understanding, ever seeking balance. Sattvic types possess a good intellect and memory, and have an inherent instinct for cleanliness and purity. Although they possess a great deal of knowledge, they always try to gain more. They have a good will towards others and allow others to prosper. They are friendly and courteous, have faith in the Divine and devotion to what is good.

Rajasic Constitution

When Rajas or the quality of turbulence prevails in a person, one is active and aggressive, but agitated and restless. Rajasic types have a nature that tries to overpower others and have a brave but jealous and sometimes cruel character. They manifest a propulsive and dynamic energy that is ever seeking and striving and which is never contented. Seldom satisfied with the positions and possessions they achieve, they are ever trying for more. They are ambitious and industrious in nature but easily become hot-tempered and egoistic, which leads to conflict and pain.

Tamasic Constitution

When Tamas or the quality of inertia prevails, a person remains trapped in negative habits and compulsions, even when they know better. Tamasic people are lazy and ignorant and do not make any real efforts to improve their condition in life. Similarly, they are not curious about things but hold to what they already know as final. Usually they are less intelligent, prefer not to work and are interested mainly in eating and sleeping. They lack cleanliness and are not health conscious. Owing to their ignorance, they are afraid of many things and do not initiate any changes on their own. For this reason they are very difficult to treat.

Mental Constitution Chart

Sattvic	Rajasic	Tamasic
Promotes knowledge by fair means	Promotes knowledge by any means	Ignorant about knowledge
Very intelligent	Average intelligence	Unintelligent
Good memory	Variable memory	Poor memory
Accepts his status and wealth; no strong desires	Strong desire for status and wealth; Ambitious and dynamic	No desire for anything, lethargic
Gives fairly to all, unselfish	Takes advantage, selfish	Selfish, non-striving
Develops purity of body, mind and speech	Agitated in body, mind and speech	Unclean in body, mind and speech
Polite, joyful	Sometimes rude and angry	Sorrowful, depressed
Calm and quiet	Brave, cruel, greedy	Fearful, vile
Believes in God or Truth	Questions God or Truth	Believes in falsehood
Inherent health and consciousness capacity	Follows health advice when convinced	Ignorant about health; does not follow medical advice
Reacts to pain and pleasure properly	Over-reacts to pain and pleasure	Fails to react to pain and pleasure

Importance of Constitution

If we observe different individuals and their nutritional requirements, their tolerance to the weather, or their behavioral patterns, we see that they have different needs for maintaining health and balance. Different people prefer different types of food, drink, and activity. Even if two individuals with identical weight and height are chosen, their requirements will still be varied. One may prefer large amounts of food or drink, while the other may prefer less. If we analyze the blood of these individuals, we may not find any substantial difference. Yet differences clearly exist. Tolerance to food, drink or environment cannot be decided by medical testing alone. It depends upon individual constitution and proclivity. By examining the Ayurvedic constitution of each individual, we can determine the food, drink, work and exercise appropriate for his or her well-being.

Each doshic type requires substances that are different from, or opposite to, their specific constitution in order to maintain health. Vata people possess qualities of coldness, dryness, roughness and lightness. Therefore, a person of Vata constitution requires food that is warm or hot, oily, soft and heavy. Otherwise, there is a tendency for Vata to increase, giving rise to Vata diseases. To compensate for Vata in the constitution, a Vata person should eat food having sweet, sour and salty tastes because these tastes possess qualities opposite to Vata.

For maintenance of health, every person should know his or her own constitution. We have seen that in each constitution there is a predominance of one or more doshas. If the daily activities, diet, occupation, and behavior are not adjusted to balance this, then the constitutional dosha will increase, giving rise to its characteristic problems. If the constitution is known, then herbs, diet, and other regimens including yoga postures can be advised both for disease treatment and to promote longevity.

Doshic Constitution Chart

Physical Features	Vata	Pitta	Kapha
Body Frame	Lean & thin	Moderate	Large & thick
Body Weight	Low	Moderate	Overweight
Skin	Dry, rough, cool, black, brown	Soft, oily, warm, fair, yellowish, red	Thick, oily, cool, pale, white, glistening
Hair	Dry, rough, brittle, blackish, brown	Soft, oily, early gray, baldness, yellow, red	Thick, oily, wavy, dark, glistening, white
Teeth	Irregular, protruded, crooked, thin gums, tendency toward tooth decay	Regular, moderate, soft gums, yellowish	Regular, strong, white, healthy
Eyes	Small, dull, attractive, brown, black iris	Medium, sharp, penetrating, green, gray, yellowish iris	Big, blue iris, thick eyelashes
Joints	Bony markings seen	Just visible	Not seen
Musculature	Slight and stiff	Medium, flexible	Firm, stout
Appetite	Variable, scanty	Good, excessive	Low but steady
Thirst	Variable	Excessive	Less
Sweating	Variable	Excessive	Less
Sleep	Scanty, interrupted	Moderate, 4-6 hrs., slightly disturbed	More than 6 hrs. sound
Taste	Sweet, sour, salty	Sweet, bitter, astringent	Pungent, bitter, astringent
Elimination	Irregular, dry, hard, constipated	Regular, soft, oily, loose	Regular, oily
Physical Activity	Fast & very active	Medium	Lethargic & slow
Sexual Vitality	Lower, variable	Moderate	Good
Pulse	Thready & weak	Jumping	Broad & slow

Doshic Constitution Chart (cont'd)

Psychological Functions	Vata	Pitta	Kapha
Dreams	Fearful, flying, jumping, running	Fiery, passionate, anger, violence, war	Watery, rivers, oceans, swimming, romantic
Emotional Temperament	Unpredictable, anxious, insecure,	Irritable, aggressive, greedy, jealous	Calm, quiet
Mind	Restless, active	Aggressive, intelligent	Calm
Faith	Changeable	Determined, fanatic	Steady
Memory	Recent good, remote poor	Sharp	Slow but prolonged
Interests	Recreation, dance, running, intellectual activities, talking	Competitive ventures, debate, politics, hunting	Family and social gatherings, cooking, collecting

ADVICE ON FOOD AND BEHAVIOR ACCORDING TO CONSTITUTION

Appropriate foods keep each dosha in balance. We will discuss these dietary factors in more detail in the next chapters.

FRUIT

VATA	PITTA	KAPHA
Sweet Fruit: Bananas, berries, cherries, coconut, fresh figs, grapefruit, grapes, mango, sweet melons, oranges, papaya, peaches, pineapples, plums	Sweet & Astringent Fruit: Apples, avocados, coconut, figs, sweet melons, sweet oranges, pears, pineapples, plums, pomegranate, prunes	Warm and Drying Fruit: Apples, apricots, berries, cherries, dry figs, mango, peaches, pears, prunes, raisins

VEGETABLES

VATA	PITTA	KAPHA
Cooked Vegetables: Asparagus, beets, carrots, garlic, cooked onions, radishes, spinach, sprouts, sweet potatoes, tomatoes zucchini	Sweet & Bitter Vegetables: Asparagus, cabbage, cucumber, cauliflower, celery, green beans, lettuce, peas, parsley, potatoes, sprouts, zucchini	Pungent & Bitter Vegetables: Beets, cabbage, carrots, cauliflower, celery, eggplant, garlic, lettuce, mush-rooms, onions, parsley, peas, radishes, spinach, sprouts

GRAINS

VATA	PITTA	KAPHA
Nutritive grains: Oats (cooked), rice, wheat	Cooling grains: Rice (basmati), rice (white), wheat	Drying grains: Barley, buckwheat, corn, millet, oats (dry), rice (basmati in small amount), rye

LEGUMES

VATA	PITTA	KAPHA
Generally avoid beans: Except mung or carefully antidote them with spices	All legumes are good: Except lentils	All legumes are good: Except kidney beans, black lentils

NUTS

VATA	PITTA	KAPHA
All Nuts are good in small quantities: Almonds, sesame, walnuts, cashews	Generally avoid nuts: Except coconut, sunflower seeds	Generally avoid nuts: Except sunflower seeds

SWEETNERS

VATA	PITTA	KAPHA
Natural sugars are good in moderation: Jaggery, raw sugar, honey	Natural cooling sugars are good in moderation: Except honey	Generally avoid sugars: Only honey and jaggery in small quantities

SPICES

VATA	PITTA	KAPHA
All spices are good with food: Especially asafoetida, basil, cardamom, cinna-mon, cumin, fennel, garlic, ginger, nut-meg, turmeric	Generally avoid spices: Except coriander, fennel, cardamom, cinnamon, cloves, turmeric and a small amount of black pepper	All spices are good: Especially black pepper, cardamom, cayenne, cinnamon, cloves, garlic, ginger, mustard, turmeric

DAIRY

VATA	PITTA	KAPHA
All dairy products are good: Buttermilk, cheese, cottage cheese, ghee, milk, yogurt	Cooling dairy products: Butter, cottage cheese, ghee, milk, paneer	Generally avoid dairy: Milk in small quantity, preferably goat's milk

OILS

VATA	PITTA	KAPHA
All oils are good: Particularly sesame, almond, ghee	Cooling oils: Ghee, coconut, olive, sunflower, soy	Take light oils in small quantities: Canola, corn, safflower, or sunflower

MEAT AND FISH

(Note: Ayurveda recommends a vegetarian diet because of its sattvic properties but describes the qualities of animal foods for those who wish to take them.)

VATA	PITTA	KAPHA
Meat is good for strengthening: Beef, lamb, chicken or turkey, eggs, seafood	Take only cooling meats: Chicken or turkey (white meat), eggs (white), rabbit	Take only lean meats: Chicken or turkey (dark meat), eggs (not fried), rabbit

LIFESTYLE INSTRUCTIONS

VATA	PITTA	KAPHA
Don't overexert or stress yourself: Avoid fasting or skipping meals; avoid strong, frequent exercise, heavy work or much travel; protect yourself from wind and cold; avoid air-conditioning; reduce stress, worry, agitation and anxiety	Don't overheat yourself: Avoid using pickles, vinegar, chilies, ketchup, carbonated drinks and alcohol; do not work late at night; avoid jobs near furnaces, fire or smoke; protect yourself from sun, heat and bright lights; avoid conflict and argument	Remain active and alert: Avoid sleeping during day time; do not eat frozen or cold food, or much sweet or oily food; do not drink ice water or soft drinks; avoid sedentary jobs, damp environments, or exposure to molds; protect yourself from cold and dampness; reduce attachments

YOU ARE PRONE TO THE FOLLOWING DISEASES

VATA	PITTA	KAPHA
Pain conditions: Nerve pain, constipation, insomnia, arthritis and joint problems, rectal prolapse, fissures on palms and soles, hysteria, epilepsy	Fever, inflammation: Hyperacidity, peptic ulcers, bleeding, skin rashes, febrile diseases, toxic blood conditions, liver disorders, hypertension	Congestion, stagnation: Diabetes, urinary stones, asthma, allergies, colds, cough, obesity, coronary heart disease, edema, benign tumors

GENERAL RECOMMENDATIONS

VATA	PITTA	KAPHA
Eat well, rich and regularly; take tonic herbs; apply sesame oil on the body and get regular massages; use medicated enemas (basti); sleep early and well	Take adequate food and liquid; donate blood; resort to water, swim; apply coconut oil to the skin; cultivate an attitude of peace and forgiveness	Eat lightly, fast occasionally; keep the mind and body light and active; apply mustard oil on the skin; take regular exercise and exert yourself; take saunas and steam baths

REJUVENATIVE MEDICINES (RASAYANAS)

VATA	PITTA	KAPHA
Ashwagandha, bala, garlic, haritaki	Licorice, shatavari, amalaki, chyavanprash, gotu kola	Haritaki, triphala, pippali, shilajit, elecampane

AGGRAVATION OF THE DOSHAS
AND THEIR MANAGEMENT

The key to Ayurvedic treatment is to know the main imbalances of the doshas and how to treat them. For this we must be able to determine the factors that aggravate the doshas, the symptoms of their aggravated states, and the appropriate counter measures to alleviate them. Below we outline these factors but will explain them in more detail later in the book.

VATA
Causes of High Vata

Vata becomes disturbed owing to cold weather, exposure to wind, or air-conditioning. Dietary factors are drinking cold substances like ice water, refrigerated foods or foods cold in energy like green salads, food that is dry, rough or light in properties like barley, millet or corn, or irregular eating habits. Excessive physical exercise, particularly of a strongly aerobic nature, as well as improper movements of the body aggravate Vata. Lack of proper nutrition and lack of proper rest are additional factors. Psychological factors that increase Vata include mental and emotional stress and anything that disturbs the peace or security of a person.

Symptoms of High Vata

High Vata is indicated by a desire for warm food, warm environment, and warm clothing. Physical symptoms are constipation, lack of energy, loss of sleep, fatigue, emaciation, abdominal distention with flatulence, blackish discoloration of feces and urine, and defective sensory functioning. Psychological symptoms arise like fear, anxiety, insecurity, confusion, and aimless talking.

Management of Vata

Vata requires patience and consistency over a long period of time in its treatment. Treatment of Vata is divided into two types based on whether the cause is tissue-deficiency (Dhatukshaya) or obstruction in the channels (Srotorodha).

The former is indicated by low body weight, while the latter is indicated by pain.

For tissue-deficiency, the best therapy is tonification or tissue-building. Anti-Vata diet should be given after making certain that the digestive fire has sufficient power to handle the heavy food required. If the digestive fire is weak, digestion-promoting herbs should be given like dry ginger, cayenne or black pepper. Then light oil massage should be given with warm oils like sesame or Mahanarayan oil, and a mild steam therapy. Herbal wines, like Draksha, can be taken before food to increase appetite, or after food as a tonic. Tonic herbs should be taken such as ashwagandha and bala. Seated yoga postures with silent meditation are helpful.

For obstruction in the channels, detoxifying and stimulating herbs such as dry ginger or fennel should be taken. Oil massage is recommended, emphasizing herbs like nirgundi or Vishagarbha oil. Special alkali medicines may be taken internally to open the channels. Mild laxatives and decoction enemas should be taken. Herbal wines prepared with jaggery and herbs like Dashamula are indicated. When the system is clean, then anti-Vata diet and tonifying methods can proceed.

PITTA

Causes of High Pitta

Pitta is aggravated by food that is hot in temperature, by spicy food like chili, black pepper, and mustard, by fried food, and by too salty or sour food. Working night shifts, in hot environments or in excessive exposure to the sun and heat increases Pitta. Prime psychological factors are anger, irritability, short temper, argument and conflict.

Symptoms of High Pitta

High Pitta brings about a desire for cooling foods, cool environment and cool clothing. Physical symptoms are excessive hunger and thirst, and burning sensations in the skin, eyes, or hands. Hypersensitivity may develop in the form of allergic rashes, fevers or giddiness. There is yellowish discoloration of the skin, eyes, urine and feces. Psychological factors of anger, rage, hatred and jealousy increase. Many inflammatory and infectious diseases can occur or problems with the blood and the liver.

Management of Pitta

Anti-Pitta diet should be taken emphasizing sweet, bitter and astringent tastes. This includes dairy products like milk, butter and ghee, mung beans, basmati rice, wheat, sweet fruit, and cool spices like coriander, turmeric and cloves. Bathing or swimming in cool water should be done, followed by light massage with cool oils like coconut or sunflower oil. Sweet aromas can be used like rose or sandalwood, or rose water can be applied to the head and nose. Purgation can be carried out in serious conditions. When Pitta has caused tissue depletion, tonic herbs like shatavari or amalaki (Chyavanprash) should be resorted to.

KAPHA

Causes of High Kapha

Kapha is aggravated by dietary factors such as cold, oily and heavy foods like yogurt, cheese, butter, milk and meat, as well as by watery fruit and vegetables like cucumber, melons, oranges, and grapes. Sweet grains like wheat and rice, particularly wheat flour, also greatly increase Kapha. Cold and damp environments or work situations are additional factors, such as working on or near water. Psychological factors are greed and attachment and unwillingness to let go of the past.

Symptoms of High Kapha

High Kapha causes digestive disorders like loss of appetite, nausea and possible vomiting, along with heaviness in the stomach. There will be heaviness in the body as a whole along with pallor of the skin, cold hands and feet, and possible swollen joints. Mucus will increase along with cough, congestion and swollen glands. One will suffer from excessive sleep, lethargy, and lack of concentration. Mentally, one feels dull, emotionally heavy and depressed, and sensory acuity gets reduced.

Management of Kapha

To reduce Kapha, one should carry out strong exercise according to one's capacity. Deep massage should be done with light and dry oils like mustard or herbal powders. Saunas should be taken or other strong means of promoting sweating. Anti-Kapha diet should be taken with dry and hot food, dominating in pungent, bitter, and astringent tastes, along with light eating and possible fasting. For increasing digestion, hot spices like ginger, black pepper, and turmeric should be used. Therapeutic vomiting can be implemented in severe cases.

4 The Ayurvedic Approach to Health

AYURVEDIC REGIMENS FOR OPTIMAL HEALTH

Ayurveda is not just a system of medicine but a science of life-quality promotion designed to increase well-being and happiness in all respects. Through Ayurvedic health regimens, we can live in such a way as to arrive at optimal health and the maximum utilization of all our faculties, which according to Yoga and Ayurveda, are unlimited. This is the great beauty of Ayurveda: It is a complete system of living physically, mentally and spiritually. It is both an art and a science, showing us not only the principles of right living but also keys to creating a style of living that makes us happy and free in all that we do.

The actual treatment of disease is a late stage of Ayurvedic treatment. Ayurvedic treatment begins with lifestyle recommendations to increase energy and promote longevity. Ayurveda prescribes complete and comprehensive health regimens from birth to old age. It shows us how we can take mastery of our own health and live the kind of lives that we really wish to. Those who take up Ayurveda find themselves carried along by a new current of energy and insight that adds a new dimension of meaning and purpose even to ordinary activities like eating and sleeping.

Maintenance of a healthy life by one's own right action is called "Swasthavritta", which means "the regimen of abiding in one's own nature." According to the Ayurvedic science of life and the yogic science of Self-realization, harmony is our natural state, while disease and sorrow are a deviation brought about by wrong actions. Yet to maintain this natural state of well being, we must know our individual nature and learn to live according to its real needs which may be different from our desires and compulsions. Ayurveda emphasizes developing our internal resources of prana and mind, rather than accumulating mere external possessions and powers as the means of fulfillment in life.

This science of self-care teaches us to live healthily and happily throughout the different stages of our lives. In order to achieve a healthy and happy life, each one of us should observe certain disciplines or duties:

• Daily regimen
• Seasonal regimen
• Occasional duties
• Observances in sexual activity
• General rules of conduct for the welfare of society
• Precautionary measures against premature aging
• Conduct and practices to achieve Self-realization

The Ayurvedic regimen of right living is designed for the achievement of a long, healthy, active life, relief from pain and disease, satisfactory enjoyment of the pleasures of life, and Self-realization. Ayurveda helps the individual to achieve the four main objectives of human life. These are Dharma, service to society; Artha, service to family; Kama, service to self; and Moksha, Self-realization. To achieve any of these goals we must be healthy, vigorous and enthusiastic.

Optimal Health (Swastha)

Ayurveda contains clear guidelines for determining the health of a person. A person whose doshas are in a state of equilibrium, who has a balanced digestion and metabolism, whose tissues and waste-materials function normally, who has acuity of the senses and a happy state of being, is a truly healthy individual. If health is maintained from birth and the three doshas remain in a balanced state, then the person achieves a well-formed body, attractive appearance, good muscular strength, and peace of mind.

Good health can be maintained until death. For this, one should intelligently follow the rules of right living according to Ayurveda. Then a person can enjoy an optimum life span of a hundred years without contracting serious diseases. He will also gain recognition in society, lasting friendships, honor and wealth because he has the energy and ability to achieve all these goals of life.

According to the ancient Ayurvedic teacher, Sushruta, the ideal healthy person is an individual that has a balanced constitution. Those who have a balanced condition from birth are able to digest the correct amount of food and maintain proper elimination. Their systems and organs function normally and they have a happy state of mind. Vagbhatta advises four rules of conduct to achieve a healthy condition of body, mind and soul:

- Only use those enjoyable objects and circumstances that your mind and senses are agreeably accustomed to;
- Do all things only after repeatedly thinking about their appropriateness for your health;
- Maintain a habit of always critiquing your own actions intelligently;
- Always use things that balance your constitution, counter the effect of the season, and enable you to maintain physical well-being.

Longevity

Vagbhatta and Charaka explain the visible physical signs of longevity at length. The skin of the individual is soft, smooth, firm, and fine. The forehead is prominent with the shape of a half-moon. The ears, when viewed from the front, appear small, but appear large, raised up, and full of flesh when seen from behind.

The eyes show their white and black parts distinctly. The eyelashes are thick and well set. The nose is straight and somewhat prominent with the end raised up and large nostrils. The lips are red but not protruding. The jaws are large, as is the mouth. The teeth touch each other and are glossy, smooth, white in color, and equal in size. The tongue is red, long, and thin. The chin is large and well formed. The nails are thin, red, and raised up slightly. The hands and feet are large, glossy, full of flesh, and reddish. The fingers are long and, when placed together, do not leave any space between them.

The back of the body is expansive and the spine well covered with flesh. The voice is deep and resonant, with a nasal sound, which lingers after speaking. The skin is glossy and vibrant. All the bones are appropriately proportioned and capable of separate and easy movement. The joints are well knit and strongly connected by muscle, strong and full of flesh. The flesh and blood are of the best quality, in the right proportion, and all the limbs are ideally juxtaposed.

Such individuals of proportionate musculature and compactness of the body possess good strength and can defend themselves from the onslaught of disease. They can withstand hunger, thirst, heat, cold, and strong physical exercise. They can digest and assimilate large amounts of food properly.

Tissue Excellence (Dhatu Sara)

Individuals with good longevity possess additional signs of their tissues being in optimal states:

- When the plasma (Rasa Dhatu) is in optimal condition, the skin is glossy, smooth, soft, attractive, thin, and tender.
- When the blood (Rakta Dhatu) is in optimal condition, all the parts of the body like the ears, mouth, tongue, lips, nose, palms, and soles of the feet are glossy and red in color.
- When the muscle tissue (Mamsa Dhatu) is in optimal condition, the back of the neck, the forehead, temples, eyes, chin, shoulders, stomach, breasts, and joints of the hands and feet

are solid, strong, attractive, and full of flesh.

- When the fat tissue (Meda Dhatu) is in optimal condition, it causes the skin to be glossy and fine, the eyes bright and attractive, the voice deep and pleasing, and the hair and nails soft and glossy.
- When the bone tissue (Asthi Dhatu) is in optimal condition, the person has large and well-formed heels, ankles, knees, elbows, collar bones, chin, and forehead. The other bones, nails, and teeth are large, compact, and steady.
- When the nerve tissue (Majja Dhatu) is in optimal condition, one possesses a soft but strong body, deep voice, glossy skin, and long and rounded joints.
- When the reproductive tissue (Shukra Dhatu) is in optimal condition, one possesses an attractive personality, joyful temperament, bright and strong teeth, hair and nails, large red lips, and a good sexual capacity.

Measurement of Body Proportion

The strength of a person's constitution can be measured by examining the proportions of the body. This is based on an individual finger unit of measurement called anguli pramana. The height of an average healthy individual is eighty-four times the finger breadth. This means that if the average finger breadth is 2 centimeters, the height should be 168 centimeters or about 5'6". The calculation of a fingerbreadth is done by taking the extent of both palms at the metacarpo-phalangial joints and dividing this amount by eight (as this width together is the average for eight fingers).

Life Span

The optimal life span of the human being is one hundred years, which is divided into three stages:

- Youth - Birth to the age of 30. This is further divided into two portions, the immature stage from birth to the age of 16, and the mature stage from 16 to 30.
- Middle age - 31 – 60 years

- Old age - 61 – 100 years

Longevity depends upon many factors but the most important is the Prakriti or birth constitution. Individuals of either Kapha or balanced constitution tend to live longer, though anyone who can manage their constitution well will have good longevity. If, in addition, the individual has good Ojas (vital energy) and excellence of all tissues (Dhatu Sara), they can live up to one hundred and twenty years. To achieve such longevity the individual should follow the disciplines described in Ayurvedic health regimens.

Physical Indications of Long Life

Charaka Samhita relates the signs of longevity, as evidenced in children:

Features Indicating Good Longevity

Hair	Discrete, soft, sparse, oily, firmly rooted, and lustrous
Skin	Thick, firm, lustrous
Head	Larger than normal in size, firmly rooted and lustrous
Forehead	Broad, strong, even, having firm union with temporal bones, and with three transverse lines, in appearance like a half moon
Ears	Thick, large in size with even lobes, equal in size and elongation downward with big ear cavities
Eyes	Equal in size, having clear cut division between pupil and sclera; strong, lustrous and beautiful
Nose	Straight, slightly curved at the tip
Tongue	Smooth, thin, red
Voice	Sweet, deep toned
Neck	Round in shape

Features Indicating Good Longevity (cont'd)

Chest	Broad and full
Hands & Arms	Round, full and extended
Thighs	Tapering downward, round and plump

IMMUNITY

Immunity is the power of the body to prevent the development of a disease or to resist a disease that has already started. This definition applies to infectious as well as non-infectious diseases. All people do not have the same resistance to disease, as we can easily observe by how different people respond to contagious diseases.

Several bodily conditions reduce immunity. Persons who are too heavy, flaccid, or fat generally have weak immune systems. Conversely, those who are too lean or thin, whose blood, bones and muscles are not well developed, who take an unbalanced diet, or who are weak or nervous, have a lower power to resist disease. Individuals with opposite qualities – who have a normal body weight, good digestion, and emotional stability – are able to resist disease. Ayurveda believes that if the body is kept healthy and its strength maintained properly, there is little chance of falling ill even to very contagious diseases.

In Ayurveda, the strength of the body has two main aspects:

• Physical strength (Vyayamashakti)
• Resistance to disease (Vyadhikshamatva)

Good quality tissues - like plasma, blood, and reproductive tissue - sufficient Kapha and good Ojas (vital energy) maintain strength and the natural resistance of the body. These are similar to the factors that promote longevity, because achieving longevity depends upon a strong immune system. Resistance to disease is classified under three main types:

- Natural – Inborn or genetic, exists from birth;
- Temporal – Under the influence of time, such as seasonal changes and the person's age;
- Developed – Produced by right action in life, like appropriate food, rest, control of sexual energy, and use of rejuvenative therapy.

For prevention of disease, Ayurveda stresses maintaining the natural defense mechanisms of the body by observing the appropriate Ayurvedic health regimens. The doshas are always in a state of flux or shifting equilibrium. They must be adjusted to ever changing environmental conditions as these factors may initiate the disease process. For maintenance of optimal health, even transient disturbances should not go unnoticed.

If a person follows the prescribed life regimen as described in Swasthavritta, he or she can attain full longevity and remain healthy throughout life. Ayurveda advises three important regimens for this purpose:

- Daily regimen (Dinacharya)
- Seasonal regimen (Ritucharya)
- Ethical regimen (Sadvritta)

AYURVEDIC HEALTH REGIMENS

I. Daily Regimen

Our daily life should consistently follow a health-promoting discipline. On this foundation, we can avoid most diseases. However, most of us do not always know what is healthy for us and varying opinions exist. Here Ayurveda puts everything into perspective. Ayurveda outlines the main practices that we should undertake on a daily basis to promote optimal health and optimal usage of our faculties.

Wake Up Time

A healthy person should arise one to two hours before sunrise. After attending to the calls of nature and drinking a glass of water, one should meditate for about half an hour and then perform some Yoga exercises including pranayama, emphasizing postures (asanas) appropriate for one's constitution as we discuss further in a later chapter on Yoga and Ayurveda.

Vata	Lotus pose, Vajrasana, Siddhasana, Alternate nostril breathing in through the right and out through the left nostril (Solar Pranayama)
Pitta	Plow pose, Shoulderstand, Shitali Pranayama or Alternate nostril breathing in through the left and out through the right nostril (Lunar Pranayama)
Kapha	Pashchimotanasana, Virabhadrasana, Neti (cleansing the nasal passages), and Agnisara, along with vigorous pranayama

Care of the Teeth

The teeth should be cleaned with medicated powders mixed with oil and salt. Alternatively, a good toothpaste can be used. The mouth is the place of Bodhaka Kapha, which allows us to taste food, and has an alkaline pH, so it should always be kept clean.

The teeth should be brushed and the gums cleaned with the fingers using powders containing astringent, bitter and slightly pungent herbs. For this purpose, a mixture of the powder of catechu, rock salt, black pepper, long pepper, camphor, turmeric, and neem in equal proportions, along with a small amount of cloves and honey is recommended.

Ayurvedic tooth powders are commercially available. They use a base of natural astringent and antiseptic clays, along with various spicy and astringent herbs in an extract form as part of the paste. If used regularly, they can eliminate many dental problems, particularly gum diseases which are the main cause of tooth loss.

Care of the Tongue

The tongue should be cleaned with a flexible strip of metal or wood. Steel or copper tongue cleaners can be purchased for this purpose. Copper also has better antiseptic properties but it tarnishes more easily than steel. Each person should use a tongue scraper every day. Clearing the tongue not only cleanses the mouth but also stimulates the whole digestive tract and improves the digestive fire. Failing to clean the tongue in the morning is considered in Ayurveda equivalent to not washing the face.

Care of the Mouth

Gargling with ¼ cup warm water mixed with a little sesame oil is good for the mouth and throat. It gives strength to the teeth, improves the voice, and imparts proper taste to the food that is eaten. It is particularly important for those with dry throats or who are prone to hoarseness, like those who speak a lot as part of their work.

Care of the Face

Every morning the face and eyes should be washed with cool water. An Ayurvedic facial paste can be made with one part amalaki powder, one-half part haritaki powder, and one-quarter part sandalwood powder. Mix this with two or three tablespoons of milk until it becomes a paste. It can be applied to the face and kept on for ten minutes and then washed off with water. This paste is astringent and helps tighten the skin and prevent wrinkling. Other herbal and facial oils can be used, such as Brahmi oil.

Care of the Eyes

Every day collyrium or kajjal should be put into the eyes. This helps remove dirt and dust, and relieves watering or burning of the eyes due to strain. Regular use of collyrium increases the brightness of the eyes and strengthens their ability to withstand bright light. Collyrium should be made from the decoction of barberry, licorice, and Triphala in equal parts along with enough honey to produce a paste. This can be applied into the eyes. If this is not available, a little ghee (clarified butter) can be put on the eyelids. Ghee counters eye infection, itch and inflammation. Various commercial kajjals are sold in Indian markets and can be used in the same way.

For making collyrium, the best substance is the ash from a ghee lamp. To make this, a copper or silver bowl with a small amount of water in it is held over a ghee lamp. The black soot that accumulates under the bowl is collected as collyrium. Medicated ghee made with the Triphala formula is also good as an oil application to the eyes.

Care of the Nose

Medicated oil should be put into both nostrils every day (this is called Pratimarsha Nasya). A few drops can be put on the end of the little finger and gently applied into the nose or, alternatively, it can be applied with an eyedropper. For this purpose, the Ayurvedic oil called Anu Tail is best or, if it is not available, such oils as sesame oil, Brahmi oil, or ghee are good. Regular use of Nasya protects the eyes, nose, and throat against disease and improves their efficiency. It helps prevent diseases of the neck and head region and strengthens the voice. It counters allergies and sinus problems and improves the functions of the mind and senses. It is probably the most important of these daily Ayurvedic health aids.

Exercise

Everyone should perform regular light exercise. This helps the body grow and become proportionate in shape and increases muscular strength. The body then can withstand exertion, fatigue, heat, and cold. The appetite is improved and health is maintained. Exercise is most beneficial in the winter and spring seasons. It is best done to the extent of half the person's exercising capacity. When sweat appears on the forehead and armpits, and respiration becomes quick and one is forced to breathe by opening the mouth, these are the signs that exercise should be stopped.

While doing exercise, due consideration must be given to age, strength, physical condition, time, season of the year, and diet. If exercise is done without paying attention to these factors and becomes excessive, then it aggravates Vata and the blood, and produces many diseases. Similarly, individuals suffering from disease or who are too old, debilitated and exhausted should not attempt strong exercise.

Western and Yogic Exercise

Yogic and Western types of exercises, when studied comparatively, have different effects. Achieving a good muscular build and power by strong working of the muscles is the aim of most Western styles of physical exercise. Yogic exercise, on the other hand, gives more importance to posture achieved and maintained with the least stressful movement. Similarly, exertions that require quick and short breathing are not recommended in Yoga. Rather, slower and longer breathing is advised because such breathing aids in longevity.

According to Ayurveda, exercise should be stopped when one has to breathe in and out quickly, when there is a sensation of dryness in the mouth, and when perspiration appears on the forehead. Exercise done with such restriction is said to be of optimal benefit. If exercise is stopped at this stage, one can prevent secretions from leaving the gastrointestinal tract and adversely affecting other bodily sites. Strong muscular exertion of the limbs can cause hepatic, splenic, or mesenteric reserves to empty themselves into the peripheral circulation. This may lead to a movement of undigested products from the digestive system into the tissues resulting in disease. Therefore, the ideal exercise according to Ayurveda is based on the understanding of central and peripheral activity of the doshas. Ayurvedic exercise emphasizes lightness of the body. Ability to flex, bend or extend is another quality that is desired. Firmness but not rigidity or hardness in the muscles and joints is the goal.

The Western style of exercise, on the other hand, emphasizes the need for "warming up", which is indicated when perspiration appears on the forehead, and does not stop the exercise at this point as Ayurveda would recommend.

Evaluation of physical ability in Ayurveda is not based on the size of the individual muscle or the "body beautiful" but the capacity to withstand heat, cold, hunger, thirst, or fatigue. Ayurveda regards Yoga as the best means of achieving the greatest physical ability. Yogic exercise also prescribes a particular diet and behaviors for the purification of body and mind, which are an essential part of optimal health and clarity of consciousness.

Smoking of Herbs

Smoking medicinal herbs (without tobacco) is useful for alleviating Kapha in the neck and head region. It is also helpful for maintaining health and treating certain diseases. Medicinal herbs used for smoking include sandalwood, cinnamon leaf, cardamom, licorice, jatamamsi, guggul, agaru, and shallaki. Such herbs should be powdered and then made into a paste and applied to a reed. This paste made into a cigarette having a thickness like the center of the thumb and the length of eight fingers' breadth. It is then dried up and the reed taken out. Then, with the help of a cigarette holder, one can smoke the cigarette after lubricating it with an oily substance like sesame oil.

Smoking can be done after taking a bath, after lunch or dinner, after brushing the teeth, after applying collyrium to the eyes, or just after getting up from bed in the morning. Smoking should not be done after drinking alcohol, when the body is too dry, or when there is a severe headache or injury to the head. Smoking should be done through the mouth and smoke should not be exhaled through the nose because this can irritate the eyes. Effects of correct and good smoking are lightness in the head, throat and chest since it liquefies excess Kapha in these regions.

Bathing

After oil massage and proper exercise, one should take a warm bath or shower. For washing the head, the water should not be too hot. A warm water bath relieves fatigue, increases strength, cleans the body, improves appetite and imparts a pleasant sensation to the body as well as the mind. The use of salts or oils in the bath water aids in moistening and nourishing the skin, as well as in relieving muscle pain and stiffness.

Showers are also good to increase sweating and reduce Kapha. However, they are more likely to deplete the bodily oils and so should be done infrequently by Vata types or those suffering from dry skin. Sesame oil can be applied before showering in order to protect the skin.

Rest and Sleep

Proper rest and sleep are essential for health and peace of mind. Before going to bed, one should practice meditation, critically examining one's own conduct. This prepares the mind for restful sleep. Usually six to seven hours of sleep gives sufficient rest to both body and mind. Kapha people may need less. Vata people may need more and can benefit from a nap during the afternoon. For Kapha people, reducing the amount of sleep is an important therapy. For Vata people, increasing sleep helps counter many diseases but it should be sleep before sunrise. Increasing sleep after sunrise generally increases Ama.

Oil Massage

Massage is an important daily or weekly practice and also has its special therapeutic value. Proper massage removes fatigue, increases muscular tone and flexibility of joints, alleviates Vata, improves circulation to the organs and the skin, eliminates waste products through the skin, stimulates the nervous system, prevents aging and increases longevity.

Oil massage is an important Ayurvedic treatment. It is relaxing to the body and mind, nourishes the skin, and improves the circulation and removes toxins. Oil massage is known in Sanskrit as *Abhyanga*. Medicated oil should be massaged on the whole body, including the head and feet. Regular oil massage removes excess fat from the skin, and makes the skin glossy, soft and strong. It protects the skin from dryness, cracking and roughness.

Persons of Vata constitution should use medicated oils prepared from demulcent herbs like shatavari, ashwagandha, or bala (like Narayana oil) and it should be applied while the oil is warm. Simple sesame oil can also be used. Regular massage is essential for keeping Vata under control. Persons of Pitta constitution should apply medicated oils using sandalwood or vetivert (like Chandabalalakshadi). Simple coconut oil can also be used. Those of Kapha constitution should use mustard or other light oils. As a result of oil massage, health is preserved, disease is prevented, and immunity increased.

Regular oil massage to the head inhibits premature hair loss or graying of the hair and promotes sound sleep. By massaging the soles of the feet and the legs, the eyesight is improved, cracks to the skin of the feet are prevented, and the reproductive system is strengthened.

Other Types of Ayurvedic Massage

Different alternative health-care systems use various substances for massage, including medicated oils, herbal pastes or powders, pieces of brick, wood, metal balls, or sand. In addition to oil massage, Ayurveda specifies four types of massage each utilizing different substances to enhance its beneficial effects.

UDVARTANA MASSAGE – Uses different ointments and powders that remove the excess oils left over on the body from oil massage. Powders of horsegram, garbanzo, or mung flour are used for this. It is a routine procedure done after Abhyanga or regular oil massage.

UDGHARSHANA MASSAGE – Uses the dry powder of herbs that provoke heat and open the pores of the sweat glands on the skin. It can also be done by using sand. Powders of calamus, lodhra, and shikai are used. Calamus is best for small children. This massage also helps to remove excess fat under the skin and reduces excess Kapha. It is one of the main treatment measures for obesity.

UTSADANA MASSAGE – Uses pieces of brick, small cuttle-fish bones, or wood sticks and has a scraping action on the skin. It is also used for removing excess oil from the skin after Abhyanga or oil massage, but has a stronger or harsher action.

ANNALEPANA MASSAGE – Is done with medicated boiled

rice. First the rice is cooked along with its husks. Then some milk is boiled along with the herbal formula Dashamula and small balls of cooked rice are put into it. These are then taken out and put in a cloth bag, with about two hands full of rice in each bag. First oil massage is done and then massage is done with rice in a downward direction, starting below the head. Massage is done on the chest, back, hands, and legs. Then the rice paste is removed and hot oil is applied again. After removing the excess oil, a hot water bath is taken.

II. Seasonal Regimen

Weather changes during the transition of seasons affect the health of all living beings. Some of these changes, such as from winter to spring, are generally beneficial, while others, such as autumn to winter, are detrimental. In order to achieve the maximum benefits from the good qualities of the atmosphere and protection from its bad effects, Ayurveda prescribes certain rules in regard to diet, behavior, and medicines called "seasonal regimen" or Ritucharya.

All activities in the universe are governed by the two energy principles of heat and cold. Based on this concept, the year is divided into two parts, accumulation (Adana) and release (Visarga). In subtropical India in which heat is the most destructive climatic factor, the accumulation phase follows the northern course of the sun (Uttarayana), the period from the winter to the summer solstice (Dec. 21 - June 21). The release phase follows the southern course of the sun (Dakshinayana), the period from the summer to the winter solstice (June 21 - Dec. 21). In the accumulation period, nature takes away energy and strength from all living beings by increasing heat and dryness. During the release period, Nature gives energy and strength back to living beings through increasing moisture and coolness. In India the monsoon begins with the summer solstice marking the transition to the period of release. Ayurvedic books explain these seasonal changes in great detail but because they apply mainly only to India, we will not go into them further here.

In the temperate parts of the world, where cold is the most detrimental factor, these two periods follow the equinoxes. The accumulation period occurs between the autumn and spring equinoxes (Sept. 21 - March 21), when increasing cold and dryness weakens the health of creatures and plants become dormant. The release period happens between the spring and autumn equinoxes (March 21 - Sept. 21), when increasing heat and moisture brings about growth and development and the production of crops.

While discussing seasonal schedules, one should understand the principle on which the pattern is based. Change in the environmental factor (hot or cold) is a stimulus for all living beings. To compensate for this stimulus, a modification in the response pattern is essential. This is called the seasonal regimen. The division of seasons depends on the actual meteorological conditions operative in each place. The substances that are advised to compensate for the effects of a particular season must be understood according to their qualities. In general, the substances to be selected in a particular season should have the opposite qualities of the season. If this rule is not followed, then there can be adverse effects.

In the hot season or summer, we should employ cooling food, herbs and lifestyle, such as fruit juices, salads and walking during the evening. In the cold season or winter, we should resort to warming food, warming herbs and lifestyle, like cooked grains and root vegetables, spices and aerobic types of exercise. In the dry season, which is generally autumn, we should take to moistening food, herbs and lifestyle, such as the use of more oils and dairy products, tonic herbs and oil massage. In the wet season, which is usually spring, we should take more drying food, herbs and lifestyle, such as dry food, spicy herbs and saunas.

Seasonal variations affect the human body and mind. Due to changes in season, changes in the doshas also take place, like accumulation, aggravation, and reduction. If the diet, mode of living and routine are not adjusted so as to keep the equilibrium of the doshas, diseases are certain to occur. The general rule is that diseases occur more during the change of seasons. We can protect against these outbreaks by the appropriate seasonal regimens.

In India there are six seasons of two months duration. Vata is provoked during the rainy season (July-August), Pitta in autumn (September-October), and Kapha in spring (March-April). Therefore, one should not take foods or do actions during these seasons that are likely to increase or provoke the respective doshas. One should resort to Vamana or herb-induced emesis in early winter, Virechana or herb-induced purgation in autumn and Basti or medicated enema in the rainy season to eliminate Kapha, Pitta, and Vata respectively. By carrying out these measures, one can prevent seasonal diseases.

In temperate climates, the Kapha season is early spring when moisture predominates, Pitta is summer, the season of heat, and Vata late autumn when wind and dryness prevail. During each season, the respective purification therapies should be employed – therapeutic vomiting for Kapha in spring, purgation for Pitta in summer, and enemas for Vata in autumn.

III. ETHICAL REGIMEN

A healthy mind is as important as a healthy body. The mind influences many physiological actions, some very strongly. When one possesses a Sattvic quality of mind, it directs all desires and actions for the welfare of an individual. Rajas and Tamas are harmful qualities of mind produced by passions and ignorant actions. Such an unhealthy mind generates wrong judgments and misconceptions, which lead to wrong actions that cause disease. Hence, every attempt should be made to increase the Sattvic quality of the mind.

Ayurveda prescribes certain rules for maintaining a healthy state of mind called "Ethical Regimen" (Sadvritta). These are not simply moral principles that reflect a particular cultural bias. They are the principles of right conduct that are applicable to all people of all times and places. Practicing them gives balance and peace to the mind. Violating or ignoring them makes us agitated in our thoughts and feelings. These are:

- Always speak the truth
- Do not lose your temper under any circumstances
- Do not get addicted to sensory pleasures
- Do not harm anyone
- As far as is possible, do not expose yourself to hardships
- Try to control your passions
- Endeavor to speak pleasant and sweet words
- Meditate every day for tranquility of mind
- Observe cleanliness in all things
- Be patient
- Observe self-control
- Try to distribute knowledge, good advice and money to others
- Whenever possible, devote your services to God, to spiritual personages, or to the elderly
- Be straightforward and kind
- Avoid irregularity in daily activities
- Consume food of Sattvic quality
- Avoid overly spicy or sour food, non-vegetarian foods and alcohol
- Behave according to the time and place where you are residing
- Act always in a courteous and polite manner
- Control your senses
- Make a habit of doing all that is good and avoiding all that is bad

General Rules of Conduct

The following principles of conduct are also generally useful for everyone:

- Avoid overeating, overdrinking, too much sexual activity, and too much or too little sleep.
- Never eat food at an unhygienic place, at an improper time, or with unhealthy people.
- Do not disclose another's faults or secrets.

- Do not take another's wealth or property.
- Do not keep company with people who break the rules of good conduct.
- Do not undertake strenuous work that is more than your physical capacity, or when you are ill.
- Do not undertake any job that is beyond your capacity.
- Control all your sense organs.

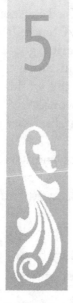

5 The Three Pillars of Life and Rejuvenation and Revitalization

The key to health can be found not in drugs or in special machines but in the prime factors on which our life and vitality is based. What we ourselves do on an everyday basis, through the factors that maintain our life, determines whether we will be healthy or sick. The three most important keys to health in Ayurveda are *food, rest* and *sexual energy*. Without proper diet, proper rest and right use of our sexual vitality, we cannot be truly healthy or vital. This is not a matter of seeing a doctor or therapist on occasion but of ourselves learning to use our energies in the right way.

On this basis, we can pursue rejuvenation and revitalization and raise our energies to a higher level of expression. Without it, our immunity and longevity must suffer. We will discuss all these factors in this chapter.

I. Food

The Ayurvedic science of diet is perhaps the most comprehensive natural system of dietetics in the world and should be examined by all that are concerned about this essential aspect of life and well being. All Ayurvedic therapies start with right diet. Food builds up the physical body; the wrong food causes disease. Food is the main pillar of our physical existence. It sustains the life of all creatures. Complexion, clarity, good voice, longevity, genius, happiness, satisfaction, nourishment, strength, and intellect are all conditioned by food in this world, as are all practices leading to liberation from this world.

Without changing our diet, even helpful herbs and exercise will not work.

Right diet can be effective for treating disease and it is certainly the best means of disease prevention. Yet most of us do not understand the qualities of foods and how to use them for optimal health.

Ayurveda divides the qualities of foods into twelve groups:

1) grains	6) salad greens	11) accessory foods
2) beans	7) wine	like oils and spices
3) meat	8) water	12) sugars
4) vegetables	9) dairy products	
5) fruit	10) cooked food	

Although Ayurveda acknowledges the food value of meat, particularly for conditions of debility, it recognizes the harm and suffering caused by eating meat as well. It tells us that we cannot escape the karmic consequences of eating meat unless it is taken to save or to protect our lives. Ayurveda also acknowledges the power of meat to breed toxins and promote diseases of both body and mind. Many modern diseases, like cancer or heart disease, are aggravated by a meat diet. Ayurveda generally recommends a vegetarian diet but lists the properties of meat for the benefit of those who take it. Generally, Vata types are more likely to feel better if they eat meat, though even for them appropriate vegetarian and herbal alternatives to meat do exist.

Wholesome or beneficial food quickly becomes one with the tissues of the body and does not aggravate the doshas. Unwholesome food, on the other hand, aggravates the doshas and damages the tissues. Wholesome food possesses a color, smell, taste and touch that is pleasing to the senses and conducive to health if taken according to the rules advocated by Ayurveda.

Best Food Articles by Type

Grains	Basmati rice
Legumes	Mung beans
Water	Rain water collected from high above ground level or spring water at a high altitude
Salts	Rock salt
Vegetables	Jivanti
Dairy Products	Ghee and milk from the cow
Oils Extracted from Seeds	Sesame oil
Animal Fats	Pig and chicken
Fruit	Grapes, raisins

Three Special Substances for Alleviating the Doshas

Sesame oil for Vata	Honey for Kapha	Ghee for Pitta

There are several other special substances:
- Amalaki is the best herb to preserve youth.
- Haritaki is the best herb for removing the doshas from the body.
- Milk strengthens life.

Properties of Food

All foods are composed of three factors:
- Five elements
- Six tastes
- Twenty attributes

A combination of two elements is responsible for producing each taste as follows:

Sweet = Earth + Water	Pungent = Fire + Air
Sour = Fire + Earth	Bitter = Ether + Air
Salty = Fire + Water	Astringent = Earth + Air

Relation of the Tastes to the Doshas

The six tastes or *rasas* represent different combinations of the five elements and either increase or decrease the doshas accordingly. For example, sweet taste is produced by earth and water elements. Hence, it increases Kapha, which has a similar nature, being composed of earth and ether.

Six Tastes and the Doshas

VATA-	Sweet, Sour, Salty	KAPHA+
KAPHA-	Bitter, Pungent, Astringent	VATA+
PITTA-	Astringent, Bitter, Sweet	
PITTA+	Pungent, Sour, Salty	

Sweet foods generally aggravate Kapha, with the exception of honey, shali rice, and barley. Usually diets of sour taste aggravate Pitta, except amalaki and pomegranate. Diets of bitter taste generally aggravate Vata and weaken sexual vitality, except guduchi. Similarly, all pungent articles except garlic and long pepper aggravate Vata and can weaken vitality unless taken as condiments with food.

Qualities of Food

Ayurveda classifies food according to twenty attributes, two pairs of ten opposite qualities:

HEAVY (Guru) – Means heavy for digestion and is connected to Brimhana or adding bulk to the tissues. All substances having sweet, astringent, and salty tastes, as well as herbs that are nutritive and restorative, aphrodisiac, and rejuvenative, are heavy. This quality belongs to the earth and water elements.

LIGHT (Laghu) – Means light in weight and easy to digest. It is linked with bringing lightness or leanness to the body. Because these substances are assimilated quickly, they provide little bulk after their absorption. Substances with bitter, pungent, and sour tastes, composed of fire, air and ether elements, like spices, are light in quality.

DULL (Manda) – Occurs in substances having a moderating energy along with cooling, calming and pacifying qualities like ghee, butter, and milk. This quality exists in earth, water, and ether.

SHARP (Tikshna) – This quality has a purifying, penetrating and stimulating affect. Pungent taste and hot energy substances like cayenne or dry ginger are sharp in their action. It is found predominantly in fire, earth, and air.

COLD (Hima) – Coldness has an astringent property (stambhana) or obstruction of motion. Bitter, astringent, and sweet substances are cold in quality, like sandalwood oil. This quality (within comfortable limits) encourages health by helping all tissues to last longer and is mainly found in the water element.

HOT (Ushna) – On the other hand, excessive heat is not helpful to the tissues, though it is useful for the digestive fire. Hot substances have the power to cause perspiration, like ginger and cinnamon. They abound in fire.

WET (Snigdha) – Oily substances like ghee or sesame oil have the property of rendering things wet (kledana). This gives them a lubricating (Snehana) effect. Oleating agents help protect the linings of the cells.

DRY (Ruksha) – Dryness has a desiccating quality that squeezes out essential material from the cells. Such substances are barley and horse gram (kulattha), or any dry food article like toast. This quality is not so useful for tissue building but helps remove excess fluids.

SOFT (Slakshna) – Means capable of holding fast. These substances have ability to heal (ropana). Only if a wound or cut is kept moist will it heal without scarring. Such soft or slimy substances avoid friction and have a soothing effect as in the cases of honey or aloe gel. It is mainly a watery quality.

ROUGH (Khara) – Means rough to the touch and has the property to remove toxins and excesses. Air-predominant substances like guggul, myrrh, and alkalis are of this quality.

CONGEALING (Sandra) – Sandra is a fluid with particles in suspension. The tissues get nourishment when a soluble solid is available for them to absorb. Such substances have the quality of binding things together like honey and sweet fruit juices.

LIQUEFYING (Drava) – Means fluids with refreshing properties that bring about hydration of the tissues. Many liquids have this property. Pure water is not useful for building tissues unless there are certain solid substances in solution or suspension. Pure water is an example of the Drava quality, but if a pinch of salt or sugar is added to it, then it becomes Sandra.

SOFT (Mridu) – Means of a pulpy quality. Fatty and oily substances are of this quality, which has a loosening effect that can be laxative. Such substances remove hardness in the body and render it soft. They contain mainly water and earth. Examples are sesame oil, ghee or any fat.

HARD (Kathina) – Ingredients in the soft and pulpy stage (Mridu) are easier to assimilate than those in a hard condition. All hard substances possess the property of making tissue firm or stable. Almonds and calcium substances like coral are hard (earthy).

FIRM (Sthira) – Means enduring and steady. All substances that are strengthening to the muscles and bones have this quality, like wheat and natural calcium.

MOBILE (Chala) – Refers to unsteady or vibrating substances. These are useful in imparting motion in a certain direction. If the sufficient time for assimilation is not available and if the movements are increased, it may result in tissue loss. All oily substances are mobile but particularly laxatives like psyllium and castor oil.

GROSS (Sthula) – Soft and round substances like butter have a covering or enveloping effect. The natural arrangement of whole substances (Sthula) is more useful than the separated or fine form (Sukshma). This is because there is a natural arrangement of bulk in gross form which aids in nutrition as well as in the excretion of waste products. This quality belongs to earth and water.

SUBTLE (Sukshma) – Alcohol, honey, and oils spread quickly in the body because of this quality. Essential oils like wintergreen or camphor and spicy herbs abound in this quality. It occurs in fire and air and particularly in ether elements.

STICKY (Picchila) – Sticky substances like the gums of different plants have the property of adhering or forming a coating which is useful for tissue building and healing. Such are gum acacia, myrrh, guggul, honey, or a demulcent oil like peanut oil.

CLEAR (Vishada) – These are substances having the power to clean. Examples are soapnut tree, shikai and such saponin-containing herbs as yucca root.

Rules for Taking Food

Ayurveda stresses the proper regimen for eating. It is not just what we eat but how we eat that matters. Eating should be done with care and with consciousness as well as for enjoyment. All individuals, even while eating wholesome food, should observe the right rules of diet.

Food should be consumed in proper quantity while it is warm and moist and it should not be contradictory in qualities. The previous meal should already have been digested. Food should be taken at a clean place in the proper company, without too much talking or laughing and with attention. The food should be consecrated with a prayer or blessing.

Warm and moist food is tastier and better stimulates the Pitta secretions (enzymes) essential for digestion. It gets digested properly and aids the downward movement of Vata (good peristalsis). Food that is slightly oily strengthens all the sense organs and increases brightness of complexion. If taken in proper quantity, it promotes longevity and does not impair the power of digestion.

While eating, due regard to one's constitution should be given and the mind should be calm and quiet. If the mind is disturbed or if there is stress and strain, then the appetite gets weakened along with the digestive nerves. Intake of food that is heavy, cold, dry, irritating or mutually contradictory in properties, or intake of food when the individual is afflicted with passion, anger or grief produces Ama (toxins), which in turn produces disease.

Indications of Proper Quantity of Food

Food is best taken in the right quantity. Even good food in the wrong quantity can cause harm. If too much food is taken, it is not properly digested and Ama or toxins are produced in the gastrointestinal tract. Right quantity of food is indicated by the absence of undue pressure in the stomach or in the sides of the chest after eating. There should be no heaviness in the abdomen or obstruction to the heart. Relief from hunger and thirst, proper nourishment of the senses, as well as a comfortable feeling while walking, talking, and sleeping and an increase in strength are additional signs that food has been consumed in the proper quantity.

Eight Factors Determining the Utility of Food

Eight factors determine the utility of food and are responsible for its beneficial effect:

1. NATURE OF FOOD (Prakriti) – Each substance has its

characteristic nature. For example, mutton is heavy, while rice is light. Sesame oil is damp and oily while toast is dry. All the qualities of food substances should be studied and applied harmoniously.

2. PREPARATION OF FOOD (Karana) – Means the transformation of food qualities through various processes like cooking, frying and roasting. Due to these processes, light substances can become heavy or vice versa.

3. FOOD COMBINATION (Samyoga) – Combination of foods may enhance the qualities of the original substances or may produce qualities other than those present in them originally. For example, the combination of fish and milk or mixing milk with sour fruit produces toxins in the blood and aggravates Pitta.

4. QUANTITY OF FOOD (Rashi) – This is of two types: Total quantity of food consumed and quantity of each particular food. Too much food or too much of any one food can cause difficulties.

5. HABITAT WHERE FOOD IS GROWN (Desha) – The place where food is grown and its variation of qualities according to the region, climate and soil are important. The negative effect of modern inorganic and chemical agricultural practices should be considered here.

6. TIME OF EATING (Kala) – This means the time when food is consumed and the state of the individual (health or diseased). While consuming food, the time of day and season should be considered. For example, heavy foods taken at night have adverse effects, as do hot foods taken in the summer.

7. DIETARY RULES (Upayoga Samstha) – These rules have already been described.

8. CONDITION OF THE PERSON EATING FOOD (Upa-yokta) – This means taking food according to one's constitution and to which one is accustomed by habitual use. The state of mind and emotions of the person are also considered here.

Wrong or Contradictory Food Usages

Various food usages are not conducive to nourishment, even if the individual food items themselves are wholesome. These are said to be contradictory usages. Such food aggravates the doshas but does not expel them from the body. It causes harmful effects because it is opposite to the qualities of the body tissues. Charaka explains seventeen types of wrong food usages. Food taken in such ways is unwholesome and should be avoided.

PLACE – Food that is wholesome for a cold region may not be good in a hot region. This is because of different geographical habitats. In deserts dry and pungent food should be avoided (as the climate is already hot and dry), while cold and oily food should be avoided in marshy areas.

TIME – Cold and dry food in winter or pungent and hot food in the summer should be avoided because the weather requires food of opposite qualities to that of the season.

POWER OF DIGESTION – Every individual possesses a specific capacity of digestion. Certain individuals do well avoiding heavy food, while others can be healthy only by consuming it. Here the difference is due to the individual capacity of the digestive fire to convert the quantity and quality of food from raw to fine materials. If we consume heavy, oily, and sweet food when our digestive power is low, for example, we will develop indigestion and toxins will form.

PROPORTION OF FOODS – For example, honey and ghee in equal proportions is not recommended.

FOOD HABIT – While advising a diet for any individual, the habitual tolerance to particular foods must be taken into account. Eating sweet and cold foods for a person accustomed to pungent and hot food may not be correct, even if the person's constitution warrants it.

ACCORDING TO DOSHA – Herbs, diet, and eating regimens with similar qualities to one's predominant dosha should be avoided, such as eating dry, cold substances or fasting when Vata is aggravated.

MODE OF PREPARATION – Although particular food items may be good, improper cooking produces negative results.

POTENCY – Mixing substances of contradictory (cold and hot) potencies together produces adverse synergism or antagonism, like taking milk with salt.

CONDITION OF THE GASTROINTESTINAL TRACT – This refers to the condition of the bowels. Taking food that is drying when there is constipation or lubricating when there is loose stool is incorrect and will cause aggravation and disease.

STATE OF HEALTH – We must consider whether the person is currently healthy or sick. For example, during convalescence from disease, a special diet is required.

ORDER – We should not eat when there are other more important bodily functions to deal with, for example, taking food before relieving an urge to evacuate the bowels.

SEQUENCE – Eating food in the wrong order, as in ingesting hot and pungent things after eating cold things or after eating ghee.

COOKING – The source of heat used for cooking food like gas, electricity, or charcoal is important. It may add to or subtract from the beneficial effects of food. Similarly, methods like slow or fast heating, direct or indirect heating or baking and roasting have different effects. Undercooking or overcooking food causes problems.

WRONG COMBINATION – Many improper food combinations exist like eating sour food with milk.

PALATABILITY – To best benefit by our food, we must have some appreciation, taste or relish for it. Eating food that is not palatable, does not smell good or causes disgust for any reason, will not produce proper nourishment.

WRONG QUALITY – Consuming substances that are not properly mature or ripe will not produce beneficial results. The same occurs if we eat over-matured, preserved or overcooked food substances.

RULES OF EATING – This means not observing the proper rules (etiquette) of eating or taking meals in the wrong company.

II. Sleep

When the body gets tired and the mind turns away from the sense organs owing to the increase of Tamas, a person falls asleep. Sleep follows a normal health pattern and brings refreshment. Deep sleep is essential for renewing both body and mind and restoring our vital energy. Without proper sleep, we will not have the proper energy to function in life. The effect of sleep is like that of diet, to provide nourishment. Just as we require proper food, so rest of the body and mind through sleep is also essential. Happiness and misery, obesity and leanness, strength and weakness, sexual vigor and impotence, consciousness and loss of sensory acuity, life and death all depend upon proper sleep.

Types Of Sleep

Sleep can be due to a number of causes. These are:

• Natural, due to exhaustion of mind and body;
• Due to increase in Tamas or dullness in the mind;
• Owing to aggravation of Kapha, which causes heaviness and fatigue;
• Caused by external injury (as to the head);
• Due to diseases and the fatigue they cause;
• Due to the advent of the night or according to the movement of time.

Daytime Sleep

Sleep during the day is usually not required unless the

person has some weakness of health or vitality. It is only recommended for those who are old, young children, persons who are exhausted (due to wounds, operation or diseases), those suffering from indigestion, diarrhea, neuralgia, asthma, or hiccups, those tired due to travel, walking, or driving, and those who have become weak due to anger and fear. It is most appropriate for Vata types. Through daytime sleep, these individuals acquire physical strength and their life span is increased.

If daytime sleep is taken when it is not appropriate, various symptoms or diseases occur. These include headache, feeling of heaviness and pain in the body, difficulty of movement, loss of movement, feeling of tightness and weakening of the heart, itching, edema, diseases of the neck and fever. Daytime sleep is contraindicated for obese persons, for Kapha constitutions, and for those suffering from Kapha diseases.

Loss of Sleep – Insomnia

Remaining awake at night aggravates Pitta and Vata and causes dryness in the body, while it decreases Kapha. Loss of sleep causes many diseases and weakens our entire functioning, adversely impacting appetite, digestion and work capacity. Loss of sleep is caused by anxiety, worry, grief, anger, fear, accumulation of stress and strain, work pressures, aggravation of Vata, excessive exercise, and increase of Rajasic quality and decrease of Tamasic quality in the mind.

To promote sleep, oil massage should be applied, particularly to the head or to the feet, and then a warm bath taken. A useful practice to promote sleep is drinking a small amount of wine and then eating some heavy food, sweets or boiled rice with milk or ghee. Singing, listening to music, joyful circumstances, the use of perfumes and flowers, or applying sandalwood paste over the forehead are also good. Good herbs for promoting sleep include ashwagandha, jatamamsi, gotu kola and valerian. Any calming meditation can be helpful as well.

III. Control of Sexual Energy — Brahmacharya

Ayurveda regards Brahmacharya as the third important Pillar of Life. Brahma means knowledge or study leading to the knowledge of God, and Charya means regimen or duty. To gain true knowledge, living a self-controlled life is essential. If the sense organs are properly controlled, the mind has clarity, good concentration and good memory. This also means controlling the sex organs, which is another meaning of Brahmacharya. Even Vatsyana, the great Indian sexologist, has mentioned in his treatise *Kamasutra* that during Balyavastha, the period from childhood until the completion of education around twenty-one years of age, celibacy should be observed. Brahmacharya is divided into three types:

• Physical – Which includes a regulated family life
• Mental – To maintain balance of mind
• Spiritual – Observing complete celibacy and practicing Yoga, rituals, and meditation for acquiring knowledge of God.

During adulthood, every healthy person possesses the desire for sexual intercourse. However, yogic teachings do not look at this act from the angle of pleasure alone. They compare the sexual act to a ritual or sacrament. This is because the person has to assume the responsibility of possibly bringing a new individual into birth. The sexual act also creates an emotional intimacy that connects people at a very deep level.

If the desire for sex is not fulfilled, it can result in physical or mental sickness, and block the person's healthy and happy functioning in life. However, excessive or perverted sexual activity results in loss of strength, weakening of immunity and disease, and disturbs the mind and heart. Only those individuals who have completely devoted their lives to spiritual practices can set the sexual desire aside without side effects because they are voluntarily sublimating this energy to a higher purpose.

Importance of Reproductive Fluids and Ojas

The reproductive fluid (shukra) is the ultimate product of nutrition in the entire body. Though the smallest in quantity of the seven tissues, it has the greatest potency. It alone of the tissues has the power to create life and to renew the body. The reproductive tissue is the only tissue that leaves the body during the normal course of activity, which makes it easy to deplete. Besides for reproductive purposes, this tissue has the additional function of providing stability to the body. Hence, undue loss of it results in loss of strength and endurance.

Ojas is extracted from the reproductive tissue and is responsible for bodily energy, brightness, strength and immunity. It is comparable to Prana, the vital force, which it helps hold in the body, providing physical and mental strength. It supports Tejas or our courage, willpower and motivation. Excessive sexual activity results in loss of the reproductive fluid and in reduction of Ojas. Therefore, efforts should be made to prevent undue wastage of these two important bodily powers, as well as to increase them through special foods and herbs, particularly when one is sexually active.

Rules for Sexual Activity

Ayurveda carefully considers the effect of season in sexual activity. During the winter season (December–March), there is less physical activity and the reproductive tissue increases. In this season, after taking Vajikaranas or aphrodisiac medicines like ashwagandha and shatavari (note section on Vajikarana), sex can be enjoyed according to one's desire. In the spring and autumn seasons (March–June and September–December), when heat and activity are moderate, sex is best every fourth day. In summer (June–September), when heat reduces the reproductive fluid, once every week or two is preferable.

Ayurveda contains special ethical and hygienic rules for sexual intercourse. Both partners should be in good physical and mental health and want to perform the act. A man should not engage in sex with a woman during her menstrual period, or with one who is devoid of passion, too old, sick, or pregnant. For the woman, the man should similarly be healthy, clean, of proper age, and passionate. Both partners, after enjoying the act, should take a cool bath and drink cool water, milk, or a little wine. They should eat food containing natural sugars. This helps restore the vital fluids.

Individuals who do not regulate their sexual impulses properly are prone to loss of strength, weak immune function, and various diseases owing to depletion of vitality. Those who regulate their sexual energy will have increased memory, power, intelligence, health, and longevity. Right use of sexual energy is a key to physical and mental health.

RASAYANA AND VAJIKARANA: METHODS OF REJUVENATION AND REVITALIZATION

Rasayana – Methods of Rejuvenation

Rasayana is a special type of treatment consisting of various methods of rejuvenation. It derives from the two Sanskrit words "Rasa" and "Ayana." The literal meaning of Rasa is the essence of something. Anything ingested into the body in the form of food or medicine is first re-synthesized into Rasa Dhatu, the basic plasma tissue that is the essence of food. Ayana is the method by which Rasa is carried to the body tissues for biochemical metamorphosis (Rasakriya). This concept of Rasayana is based upon the two principles of conservation and transmutation of energy. It preserves our vital energies so that they can increase to the point at which they can bring about an inner transformation or revitalization.

Rasayana therapy strives to improve physical, mental and ethical qualities. It inhibits old age, restores youthfulness, improves the complexion and the voice, and increases physical strength and immunity. It strengthens memory and intelligence, gives happiness, and promotes a life that is beneficial to others.

Every individual has a natural life span of about one hundred years. This life span is nothing but the combined effect of the reserve force of all organs, tissues and systems. This reserve force has six components:

1. Maternal influence	2. Paternal influence	3. Nutrition
4. Subtle body	5. Soul	6. Congenital factors

Hereditary and parental factors, which are largely genetic, combine with subtle factors that are karmic or from past life influences. To this is added the nutrition throughout life. The genes are like physical karmic patterns, while the subtle body represents the mental karmic patterns. The individual soul is the reincarnating entity behind the entire process and its particular level of development.

If the optimum use of this reserve force is made, one can achieve one's full life span. On the contrary, inordinate use of the sexual organs, improper food and rest, a reckless approach to the problems of life, and accumulation of stress and strain consumes the reserve force resulting in a shorter life span. These result from not living in harmony with our soul and with our karma. Therefore, individuals having a sattvic mind, who follow ethical living practices, are in the best position to achieve the benefits of Rasayana.

Preliminary Practices

In order to achieve the maximum benefit, the body must be made sensitive and receptive in order to assimilate the Rasayana medicine. This is just like how dirty clothes cannot be properly re-colored unless their dirt is first removed. The same is the case with the human body. Unless toxins are first eliminated, the body cannot be rejuvenated.

Preliminary to Rasayana, Pancha Karma or the Five Purification Practices are usually performed (see Chapter II.5). Such practices aim at removing waste products and aggravated doshas from the body. They also eliminate toxins (Ama) which are accumulated in the tissues and make the body receptive to rejuvenating methods.

An appropriate ethical regimen is necessary during Rasayana treatment to assure the proper rejuvenation of the mind to go along with that of the body. These are rules similar to the Yamas and Niyamas, the ethical practices of the Yoga system, like nonviolence and contentment. The person who follows these rules achieves a steady and tranquil mind. This results in the withdrawal of the sense organs from disturbed activity and complete concentration in the Self, so that there is a minimum expenditure of life energy. When this basal energy is converted into higher forms by the practice of Yoga, it improves all higher brain functions.

The effects of Rasayana therapy are better achieved if the individual is not too old (before the age of seventy), has a healthy body and mind, possesses good tolerance for physical and mental pain, is kind, compassionate and even-tempered.

How Rasayana Acts

The actions of Rasayana regimens are manifold:

- To increase body tissues
- To increase digestive power
- To increase the metabolic process at a tissue level or to improve endocrine function
- To remove waste products or to remove excess tissues in the body
- To increase the functional capacity of the brain
- To increase the strength and immunity of the body
- To destroy disease and establish homeostasis of energy, which prevents early aging

Types of Rasayana

There are two basic types of Rasayana therapy according to the place wherein the treatment is given:

- Allowing Movement or Ambulatory - Vatatapika
- Requiring Inaction or Non-ambulatory - Kutipraveshika

    Rasayana therapies are differentiated according to their purpose:

- For a specific purpose (Kamya)

- For improving longevity (Vayasthapana)
- For improving brain function (Medhya)
- For improving action of the tissues
- For improving action of the channel systems
- For improving action of the senses
- To counteract a particular disease (Naimithik)
- Daily Rasayana (Ajasrik)

Kutipraveshika Rasayana

Of these above types, the non-moving type of Rasayana is the most effective and gives the maximum benefits. This requires that the patient stays in the same place throughout the treatment and avoids all physical movement as much as possible. A special type of building is constructed for this purpose, called a three-walled hut (Trigarbha Kuti). The idea behind its construction is that the person inside it should not come into contact with the heat of the sun or dry wind, which take away vitality. If possible, air-conditioning and weatherproofing should be done to eliminate heat and drafts. The room should have all required medicines and amenities necessary for daily life.

The person who undertakes this special type of rejuvenation treatment should enter the building on an auspicious day after his body and mind have been purified by the necessary Pancha Karma practices and the correct ethical regimen. He should stay in this room for up to three months. During this period, he should avoid contact with the outside world and keep clear from negative thoughts and emotions. To maintain tranquility of mind, he should perform meditation, Pranayama, and other Yoga practices. During this Rasayana period, he should eat only Rasayana substances that have been prescribed by his Ayurvedic doctor and not take any other foods.

For Kutipraveshika, Rasayana formulas containing complex herbal drugs, called Divya Aushadhi or "herbs having spiritual effects", are prescribed. Such are Brahma Rasayana, Chyavana Prash and herbs like gotu kola (brahmi), bhallataka, shilajit, and long pepper (pippali).

Ambulatory (Vatatapika) Rasayana

This type of Rasayana can be done while engaged in daily activities, though one should reduce these and have more time for relaxation and meditation. Although of less benefit than the previous method, it is suitable for everyone. However, one should not eat oily, fatty, sour or spicy food during this time. A sensate life style and the drinking of alcohol should be given up. All the Rasayana substances mentioned for the previous method can be used.

General Rasayanas

For promoting longevity, retarding the aging process, and prolonging youthfulness, herbs like amalaki or guduchi are advised. These can be taken like food supplements as general Rasayanas.

For increasing the capacity of the brain, herbs that provide nutrition to the brain centers are indicated. These help increase intelligence, memory, and quick comprehension. Herbs like calamus, shankha pushpi, jatamamsi, brahmi, and manduka parni are the best rejuvenatives for the brain (Medhya Rasayanas). They accelerate the development of the faculties of the higher brain centers.

For specific tissues, certain herbs and foods function as Rasayanas. Some of these are:

Rasayanas for the Tissues

1. Plasma (Rasa)	Draksha, shatavari, dates
2. Blood (Rakta)	Amalaki, lauhadi rasayana, bhringaraj, suvarna makshika
3. Muscle (Mamsa)	Masha, ashwagandha, bala, nux vomica, silver bhasma
4. Fat (Meda)	Guggul, shilajit, haritaki, guduchi, garlic

Rasayanas for the Tissues

5. Bone (Asthi)	Shukti (mother of pearl) bhasma, prawal (coral) bhasma, kukkutanda bhasma, mrigash-ringa bhasma, vamsharochan, prishnaparni
6. Nerve (Majja)	Calamus, gotu kola, shankhapushpi, loha bhasma, gold bhasma, makaradhwaja
7. Reproductive (Shukra)	Kapikacchu, vidarikanda, shatavari, ashwagandha, ghee and milk

Just as for the tissues, different herbs and foods function as Rasayanas for the different channel-systems. The Rasayanas for the other channel-systems are the same as those for their respective tissues.

Rasayanas for the Bodily Systems

Respiratory	Chyavan prash, vardhaman pippali (long pepper), vardhaman marich (black pepper)
Digestive	Long pepper, bhallataka, haritaki, suvarna parpati
Water metabolism	Fresh ginger, cyperus, cardamom
Urinary system	Punarnava, gokshura
Excretory system	Kutaj, vidanga, triphala
Sweating system	Basil, nux vomica, datura

Vardhamana Rasayana is a special method by which tissues in the body are saturated with a particular medicine by unit increase and unit decrease method. For Vardhamana Pippali, take one-half cup of water and one-half cup of milk, add one long pepper (pippali) on the first day, and boil until the water evaporates, and drink the milk. On successive days, add one additional pippali until the total amount reaches the number of seven, nine, or eleven. Then reduce the amount taken each day by one until the amount of one long pepper is again reached. This cycle should be repeated for three months. For Vardhamana Marich (black pepper), start with two black pepper corns and increase the amount by two. Go up to sixteen, eighteen, or twenty pepper corns and gradually reduce the amount again to two, also for a three month period. This is a slow method of rebuilding the lung tissue, which does not damage the lungs and increases their energy in a way that persists for a long period of time.

Rasayanas for the Organs

Eyes	Triphala, licorice, shatavari
Nose	Nasya of Anu Tail
Skin	Tuvarak, catechu, bakuchi
Brain	Gotu kola (brahmi), calamus
Heart	Guggul, elecampane, gold bhasma
Liver	Aloe, guduchi
Neuro-Muscular System	Bala, nagbala, garlic, guggul

Rasayanas According to Constitution

Vata	Bala, ashwagandha, shankha pushpi
Pitta	Amalaki, shatavari, guduchi, gotu kola
Kapha	Bhallataka, guggul, long pepper, garlic

Vajikarana – The Use of Aphrodisiacs

Charaka states that every human being possesses three basic innate urges or drives: The instinct for self-preservation, the instinct to gain wealth, and the instinct for self-realization. The desire to have children is the attempt to fulfill the first of these three desires, that of preserving life. Although the science of Vajikarana attempts to increase sexual power, its real aim is genetic improvement. It has been clearly stated that those who are unable to control their sexual urge should not use these medicines. This method should be adopted after the person attains the age of puberty and when hormones and secondary sex characteristics have developed. It should not be used before the age of sixteen and after the age of seventy. Like Rasayana, purification of body and mind are essential for achieving the maximum benefits of Vajikarana.

Differences Between Rasayana and Vajikarana

Rasayana	Vajikarana
Advisable for male and female	Needed mainly by men (Woman herself is the best Vajikarana)
Useful in all age groups	Should not be used before sixteen or after seventy
Can be used to eradicate certain diseases	Not useful to eradicate diseases
Sexual contact to be avoided	Sexual enjoyment with restraint
Aim is to prepare for healthy self-realization	Aim is to fulfill urge to preserve life through good progeny
Medicines are composed of all five elements	Predominantly earth and water elements

Vajikarana Medicines

In many Vajikarana preparations, the eggs of different birds, the flesh of various animals (including birds and fish), shellfish like shrimp and oysters, as well as milk, honey, ghee, and sugar are used. Traditional Chinese medicine uses similar items. Again the yogic precautions against meat and eggs should be taken into consideration. Similarly, the following foods and herbs are useful:

Vajikarana Foods	Cane sugar, milk, ghee, masha, urad dal, almonds, cashews, sesame seeds, garlic, onions
Vajikarana Herbs	Shatavari, ashwagandha, kapikacchu, licorice, saffron, bala, mahabala, vidarikanda, gokshura, meda, kokilaksha, kakoli

Taking such herbs and foods when one is sexually active not only guards against undue loss of energy but also increases sexual enjoyment. Many of them help produce a superior quality reproductive fluid for those aiming at producing good genetic quality in their children. These same items are generally good for revitalization during conditions of debility.

PART TWO

Methods

of Ayurvedic

Treatment

6 Ayurvedic Herbology

E very system of medicine uses various substances to promote healing. Modern medicine employs mainly chemical drugs, while
natural systems of healing rely on food and herbs. Ayurveda
uses all the healing substances that nature provides and gives
us a special energetic language in which we can understand
their properties. It has a comprehensive system for utilizing all
the healing powers of all things. Ayurveda enables us to use all
the bounty of nature for healing our bodies, minds and souls.

The Ayurvedic science of healing substances or Ayurvedic
Pharmacology is called Dravyaguna Shastra or the science of
substance and quality. It classifies substances (Dravya), their
properties (Guna), and actions (Karma) in an interrelated manner. This science deals with all aspects of herbal and mineral
medicines such as identification, usage, dosage, and methods
of processing. While using a variety of minerals, Ayurveda is
still primarily an herbal medicine and relies upon herbs for the
majority of its treatments.

To prescribe medicines, we must have an adequate theory
about their qualities and how they relate to the human being.
Ayurveda prescribes medicines based upon the law of unifor-
mity in Nature. According to this law, healing substances and
living bodies are similar in composition, both being products
of the same cosmic forces. Herbs influence the body according

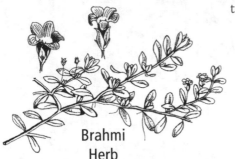

**Brahmi
Herb**

to their nature and attributes. Substances of opposite attributes serve to correct conditions of imbalance. This is the main approach used in Ayurvedic healing.

All substances in the universe are composed of different combinations of the five great elements. Because the human body is composed of these same elements, all substances can be used as medicines when we apply them according to their elemental constituents to counteract the imbalances of the elements within the body. Ayurvedic Herbology has several branches:

Branches of Ayurvedic Herbology

- Ayurvedic Pharmacognosy – The identification of medicinal substances according to their name and form. This provides various classifications of herbs and their morphological character, or botany.
- Ayurvedic Pharmacology – The science of the properties and actions of medicines. It classifies medicines according to their energetics as defined by Ayurveda.
- Ayurvedic Pharmaceutics – The Ayurvedic technology of preparing medicines including decoctions, powders, pills, tablets, herbal wines and oils. It also deals with the collection and storage of herbs.
- Ayurvedic Therapeutics – the science of employing medicines Ayurvedically. It indicates how to use medicines to treat diseases, including dosage, time of ingestion and mediums for taking, as well as the sites in the body at which the herbs are introduced.

Ayurvedic Medicines

1. Food	2. Medicine	3. Poison

Charaka classifies healing substances into three groups: Substances useful for tissue building like wheat, rice, and milk are regarded as foods. Substances which, after entering the body, get eliminated through the gastrointestinal tract within a specified period after their corrective role is over are medicines. This includes most herbs, which affect bodily processes, such as the increased sweating that comes through hot herbs like ginger, but which do not function as foods for directly building tissue. Poisons are harmful to the tissues and get stuck within them, causing many harmful effects. The accumulation of such toxic substances decreases the functional capability of the entire body, as we are witnessing today with various forms of heavy metal toxicity in our polluted environment.

Some overlap exists between these three categories. Some foods have medicinal effects, like the action of barley to increase urination. Some herbs, particularly tonics like ashwagandha, have tissue-building action like foods. Poisons have limited medicinal action in acute conditions, such as for stopping pain.

By this theory, all chemical drugs are poisons and must have side effects. Ideal or safe medicines are those that leave the tissues after their actions are over without causing any harm. An ideal medicine should have four qualities:

• It should be easily available.
• It should have the necessary power to eradicate the disease.
• It should have no side effects if taken in the right preparation.
• It should contain all the appropriate qualities of taste, energy and post-digestive effect to produce the desired effect.

Ayurvedic Classification of Medicines

The Ayurvedic understanding of herbs is profound and many-sided. It considers all aspects of how an herb is prepared and used. Ayurveda classifies herbs in various ways according to their usage, energetics, origin and action on the doshas. All these factors must be properly considered before an herb is chosen for treatment.

Power of Herbs

Herbs may be strong in potency like bhallataka (marking nut), which causes severe allergic reactions, or aconite, which is poisonous. They may be medium in potency, which includes most herbs of bitter, pungent, or astringent tastes like cayenne, golden seal or white oak bark, that have strong short term action and potential irritant effects. Or they may be mild in potency and safe for long-term usage, such as tonics like amalaki, licorice or marshmallow, which can function as foods or as food supplements. However, all herbs have indications and contraindications that must be considered for proper usage.

Source of Derivation

Substances vary in quality according to the nature of their origin, which is twofold as organic and inorganic. Organic substances derive from either animals or plants. Animal sources are mammals (born from wombs), birds and fishes (born from eggs), insects (born from moisture), and worms (born from the earth). Plant sources are large trees with fruit but no apparent flowers (vanaspati) like tropical fig trees; medium trees with both fruits and flowers (vriksha) like mango or citrus; shrubs and small plants (virudha); herbaceous plants and grasses (oshadhi).

Inorganic sources are mainly minerals that can be gathered from mines, mainly in mountain regions, but others are also available from the desert, from the sea, or wherever they happen to be found.

Energetics

Ayurveda categorizes all healing substances according to a unique system of energetics, which is one of the most important and effective aspects of this wonderful system. It considers elemental constituents, taste, potency, post-digestive effect and special action, which are explained below. This is the main Ayurvedic method of understanding herbs.

Action on the Doshas

The doshas are the main focus of Ayurvedic treatment and herbs are classified relative to them as well. Medicines have their specific effects on Vata, Pitta and Kapha. They serve to pacify, purify, disturb or harmoniously maintain them. All of these actions are necessary at some stage of treatment. The action of herbs on the doshas is generally an extension of their energetics.

The Five Great Elements in Herbs

The five great elements are responsible for the formation of the universe and the human being. They are the keys to helping us understand herbs as well as bodily processes. Their properties

Elemental Correspondences	Properties	Effects
EARTH - Smell, sweet, slightly astringent in taste	Cold, wet, slow, heavy, immobile, solid, hard	Promotes growth, weight gain, compactness of tissues, stability, strength, downward flow of Prana (elimination)
WATER - Taste, All tastes, mainly sweet	Cold, wet, slow, heavy, mobile, liquid, soft, sticky	Moistening, oleating, binding, holding in solution, pleasing
FIRE - Sight, Pungent, slightly sour and salty	Hot, sharp, subtle, rough, hard, light, clear	Warming, digestive stimulant, gives luster, improves complexion, gives illumination, causes tears, burning, moving upwards (emetic, expectorant)
AIR - Touch, Astringent, slightly bitter	Subtle, hard, cold, light, clear, mobile	Cleansing, gives lightness, roughening, agitating
ETHER - Sound, no taste	Loosening, subtle, soft, penetrating, discriminating, softening, increases porousness	Opens the channels, imparts lightness

and actions are as follows:

The effects of natural substances are determined by their constituent elements. Earthy substances are hard, solid, and dense, or soft, moldable, and shapeful in qualities. They emit smell or fragrance when rendered to powder form. Watery substances have a certain amount of fluid that can be judged by the juice or water content within them. Fire-dominant substances are easy to crush, emit a strong odor and possess a bright color. A substance with dusky colors and having a thin, hard, patchy structure as well as a rough texture is air-dominant. Ether-dominant substances are porous, easy to compress and disintegrate but do not exhibit color or odor.

THE ENERGETICS OF HEALING SUBSTANCES

The most important Ayurvedic method of classifying medicines is according to their energetics, which consists of related factors:

1. Taste-Rasa	2. Post-digestive effect- Vipaka	3. Energy-Virya	4. Special action-Prabhava

1. TASTE – RASA

What are the different tastes possible for us to experience and what are their properties. Ayurveda recognizes the existence of six tastes or rasas (essences) – sweet, sour, salty, pungent, bitter and astringent. Each of these is composed according to a preponderance of two of the five elements. The appropriate diet and herbs are selected according to the elements that match those of the dosha to be treated.

Taste and Aftertaste

Each substance in the physical world is composed of all five elements, though one element may predominate. Hence, it is impossible to find a substance having only one taste. When a substance is called sour, for example, this does not entirely exclude the other tastes. It means that the sour taste is predominant, while the other tastes are secondary. These second-ary tastes can manifest as aftertastes (Anurasa). The taste is perceived immediately, while the aftertaste (Anurasa) arises later only after the taste has already been noted. For example, the Ayurvedic compound Triphala has a powerful astringent taste but leaves a sweet aftertaste in the mouth that can be perceived by drinking water after having taken the herb which will then taste sweet.

Formation of the Tastes from the Elements

ELEMENTS	TASTES
Ether+Air	Tikta - Bitter
Air+Fire	Katu - Pungent
Fire+Water	Lavana - Saline, salty
Water+Earth	Madhura - Sweet, plain taste
Earth+Fire	Amla - Sour
Earth+Air	Kashaya - Astringent

For building bodily tissues, earth and water elements are the most useful because they increase bulk and bodily fluids. Sweet, sour, and astringent tastes, possessing earth and water elements to some degree, are good for this purpose. Sweet taste is the strongest because it is composed entirely of earth and water, which is why sweet is the main taste found in foods. Sour taste is second in nutritive properties and is thirst-relieving. Astringent taste works more to preserve than to build the body fluids because it has a holding or protecting action.

On the other hand, substances having bitter, pungent, and salty tastes, predominating in fire and air elements, are used mainly to reduce bodily tissues and for eliminating toxins. Bitter taste is strongest in this regard because, being composed of air and ether, it reduces all the heavier elements. Pungent is second and has the capacity to burn away the heavier elements with its fire content. Salty taste also has some water-preserving action as well as an ability to burn up toxins, so it has both building and reducing qualities.

Inference of Taste from Plant Characteristics

We can infer the taste of a plant from its botanical characteristics. Plants that exhibit fully developed features including roots, stem, branches, leaves, flowers, and seeds or fruit, usually possess a pleasant or sweet taste and are useful for nourishment. Most fruit trees are of this type. Their earth and water elements give them a complete development as plants, which in turn promotes their nutritive qualities.

Plants that are long living, bulky, and hard usually have an astringent taste, as this taste derives from earth and air elements. Many non-flowering trees have this taste in their leaves, such as oaks or maples. Although sour taste derives from earth and fire elements, plants yielding sour taste contain less bulk and need support to stand, like citrus trees or berries.

As pungent taste is formed by fire and air elements, plants possessing this taste do not have hard or well-formed characteristics, nor do they contain any juice. But they usually have bright colored flowers and often have aromatic volatile oils, like mints and sages. Few plants have a salty taste, as this derives from fire and water. Mainly seaweeds come in this category, but it occurs as a secondary taste in some desert plants, as well as coming from mineral salts. Bitter taste is formed by ether and air elements. Plants yielding bitter taste are light and lacking in bulk like aloe, barberry or golden seal. However, some slender and small trees, like willow and aspen, possess this taste as well, often with some astringency as well. This combination of astringent and bitter tastes is probably the most common taste in plants.

Classification of the Six Tastes

We can discriminate the actions of the six tastes by three prime sets of qualities:

- damp/dry
- hot/cold
- heavy/light

Damp and dry refers to increasing or decreasing bodily fluids. Sweet taste is the dampest taste, followed by salty and sour. For this reason, sweet, sour and salty beverages, like lime juice with sugar and salt, are good for preventing dehydration. Pungent taste is the driest taste, followed by bitter and astringent. Astringent taste is generally drying but helps preserve bodily fluids.

The six tastes are classified into two groups according to their heating and cooling properties:

Sweet	Damp, cold, heavy	Sour	Damp, hot, light
Saline	Damp, hot, heavy	Pungent	Dry, hot, light
Bitter	Dry, cold, light	Astringent	Dry, cold, heavy

- Fiery tastes: Pungent, Sour and Salty - increase the digestive power and Pitta;
- Cooling tastes: Sweet, Bitter and Astringent - decrease digestive power and Pitta.

Hot and cold means increasing or decreasing bodily heat, particularly the digestive fire as well as Pitta dosha. Pungent is the hottest taste followed by sour and salty. For this reason, spices and condiments that stimulate the appetite are predominantly pungent (spicy), sour and salty in taste. Bitter is the coldest taste, followed by astringent and sweet. Bitter, astringent and sweet herbs are good for countering fever and inflammation.

Heavy and light means increasing or decreasing bodily tissues. Sweet is the heaviest of the six tastes followed by sour and salty tastes. These are the three main tastes found in foods and have building or tissue-increasing properties. Bitter is the lightest taste, followed by pungent and astringent. These are the three tastes least common in foods and are used mainly for detoxification purposes.

Relation of Tastes and Doshas

We have observed that the six tastes represent six different combinations of the five great elements and their resultant activity. For example, as sweet taste is produced by earth and water, it increases the earthy and watery elements of the body, which are the main elements that compose Kapha dosha. Conversely, it decreases the opposite components of ether, air and fire elements, the constituents of Pitta and Vata.

Sweet, sour, and salty tastes, predominating in earth and water, increase Kapha, while pungent, bitter and astringent tastes, which predominate in ether, fire and air elements, reduce it. Conversely, sweet, sour and salty tastes, predominating in earth and water, decrease Vata while pungent, bitter and astringent tastes, which have more air and ether components like Vata, increase it.

Pungent, sour, and salty tastes, possessing fire, increase Pitta, while bitter, astringent, and sweet tastes, which have no fire, reduce it. In this manner, the six tastes increase or decrease the doshas in a regular manner. But to accomplish this aim, the herb or food must first pass through the digestive process. This aspect is dealt with under post-digestive effect.

Actions of the Six Tastes

SWEET TASTE – Has the same nature as the body, increasing bodily tissues including plasma, blood, muscle, fat, bone, nerve and reproductive. It prolongs life, nourishes the sense organs, imparts vigor and improves the complexion. It has a lubricating effect on the skin, hair and voice and promotes strength. Psychologically, it promotes cheerfulness, energy and happiness, containing the energy of love.

Sweet taste increases Kapha and decreases Pitta and Vata. It is cold, damp and heavy for digestion, reducing Agni. Excess use of the sweet taste produces such Kapha disorders as obesity, lethargy, heaviness, loss of appetite, edema, dyspnea, cough, cold, constipation and vomiting.

SOUR TASTE – Increases appetite, promotes salivation, stimulates digestive power and regulates peristalsis. It conducts the food downward in the gastrointestinal tract, moistens it, and aids in its proper absorption. It promotes strength, builds up bodily tissues (except the reproductive) and provides nutrition to the heart. It awakens and stimulates the mind and senses.

Sour taste decreases Vata but increases Pitta and Kapha. It is light, hot and oily in character. Excessive use of sour taste produces thirst, dissolves Kapha, increases Pitta, causes acidity, makes the blood toxic, damages the muscles, mucus membranes and teeth, renders the body tissue loose and produces edema in emaciated persons.

SALTY TASTE – Improves digestion, imparts relish to food, removes obstructions in the channels, is laxative, reduces stiffness and softens accumulations. It overpowers the other tastes, increases secretions in the mouth and liquefies mucus (is decongestant).

Salty taste decreases Vata but increases Pitta and Kapha, is neither very heavy nor very oily and is hot. Excessive use of salty taste aggravates Pitta, vitiates the blood and provokes thirst. It weakens the muscles, aggravates skin rashes, increases toxins, destroys virility and impairs the function of the nervous system. It can induce premature wrinkles on the skin, cause gray hair and baldness.

PUNGENT TASTE – Purifies the mouth, imparts relish to food, stimulates digestion and helps destroy bacteria and parasites. By its hot nature it causes sweating, running of the nose and watering of mouth and eyes. It helps to reduce edema and obesity and removes excess oiliness in the body. It eliminates excretory matter, decreases itching, breaks stagnation of the blood, removes obstructions and opens the channels. It stimulates the mind and senses and clears the head and throat.

Pungent taste decreases Kapha but increases Pitta and Vata. It is light, hot and dry in character. It irritates the mucus membranes and can cause skin rashes. Excess use destroys virility and gives rise to emaciation. It produces fainting, choking, giddiness and burning sensations. It diminishes strength and increases thirst.

BITTER TASTE – Although it produces an unpleasant taste in the mouth, it has an appetizing action and cleanses the digestive tract so that the digestive fire can function better. It counters fevers, is detoxifying, removes poisons and destroys parasites. It relieves burning sensations, itching, thirst and inflammatory diseases of the skin. It imparts firmness to skin and flesh, reduces obesity and removes excess water from lymph, sweat, urine, feces, bile and mucus membranes.

Bitter taste decreases Pitta and Kapha but increases Vata. It is dry, cold and light in character. Excessive use produces dryness, loss of strength, tissue depletion and generates various Vata disorders. It can weaken the appetite and cause thirst and diarrhea. It is mainly used short term for its medicinal values and is seldom taken in quantity.

ASTRINGENT TASTE – Has styptic and healing properties and promotes the healing of wounds, cuts, sores and injuries. It purifies the blood, counters toxins and removes an excess of watery waste products from the body. It counters bleeding, stops sweating, stops cough and stops diarrhea.

Astringent taste decreases Pitta and Kapha but increases Vata. It is dry, cold and heavy in character. Excessive use produces dryness in the mouth and skin, constricts the channels, obstructs speech and produces gas in the stomach and intestines. It inhibits the excretion of feces, urine, and sweat, causing a build-up of waste-materials in the body, prompting various Vata diseases.

Action of the Tastes on the Tissues

Herbs work to increase or decrease bodily tissues according to their tastes. Only two tastes – sweet and sour – serve to regularly increase bodily tissues, providing direct nutrition for the tissues. Sweet taste increases all bodily tissues, while sour taste increases all except reproductive tissue. For this reason Ayurveda does not recommend sour taste for conditions of infertility or sterility.

The other four tastes – salty, pungent, bitter and astringent – generally decrease bodily tissues. Salty and astringent tastes can help preserve bodily fluids and so, in the proper amount, help maintain tissues. Pungent taste stimulates appetite and digestion that leads indirectly to tissue growth, so along with foods, can have a building effect. Bitter is the most depleting of the tastes, but by removing toxins can aid in long term growth.

Actions of the Tastes on the Waste-materials

Herbs work to facilitate or inhibit the elimination of waste-materials. The earth and water dominant group – sweet, sour, and salty tastes – facilitates the movement of waste-materials by their heavy and moist nature. They are laxative, carminative (dispel gas), and increase urination. The air dominant group – pungent, bitter, and astringent tastes – inhibits the formation and movement of waste-materials and causes flatulence or constipation, owing to their drying nature.

Action of the Tastes on Agni (The Digestive Fire)

The different tastes work to increase or decrease the digestive fire and regulate metabolism. Fiery tastes – pungent, sour, and salty – naturally increase Agni, promote appetite and burn Ama or toxins. Bitter taste, although cold in nature, stimulates Agni by promoting Samana Vayu or the digestive nerves. Sweet and astringent tastes decrease Agni by their heavy and constricting nature.

Action of the Tastes on the Channel Systems

The channel systems of the body, from the digestive system to the channels of the mind, are a key to health. Only if the energy in them is flowing smoothly will we feel well. To keep this energy moving properly, we must understand how the six tastes affect them. Pungent, bitter and salty tastes, by their penetrating natures, help clear the channels. Sweet, sour and astringent tastes tend to clog or block the channels.

Pungent taste, by its air and fire constituents, absorbs fluid and expels obstructive material in the channels, promoting circulation. Bitter taste reduces toxins and, because of its subtle nature, permeates even to the minutest channels, relieving obstructions. Salty taste liquefies solids, removes congestion and has a laxative action.

Sweet, sour, and astringent tastes have no such cleansing effects. Sweet taste creates heaviness that obstructs the channels. Sour taste aggravates inflammation in the channels. Astringent taste, by its constricting nature, blocks the movement of substances within the channels.

2. POST-DIGESTIVE EFFECT – VIPAKA

The digestive fire acts upon any herb or food ingested. During the process of digestion, the six tastes (Rasas) are re-synthesized into the three post-digestive effects (Vipaka) sweet (Madhura) Vipaka, sour (Amla) Vipaka, and pungent (Katu) Vipaka. Though post-digestive effect is explained in the terminology of the tastes, it cannot be sensed by the tongue and occurs at an internal organic level.

Post-digestive effect is inferred from the final action of the ingested food or medicine. There are two main effects of the digestive process – building or reducing - anabolic or catabolic (brimhana and langhana in Sanskrit). For this reason, Sushruta classifies post-digestive effect into two types only – heavy (building) and light (reducing). However, Charaka classifies them according to their effect upon the doshas – sweet, sour and pungent – or as relating to Kapha, Pitta and Vata. Out of these three, sweet is the same as heavy, while sour and pungent are included under light. Post-digestive effect occurs mainly in the field of Apana Vayu, the downward moving Prana in the large intestine, which reflects the ultimate result of digestion.

• SWEET POST-DIGESTIVE EFFECT is the result of sweet and salty tasting food and herbs. It decreases Pitta and Vata but increases Kapha. It aids in the smooth elimination of feces and urine, and increases the reproductive fluid.

- SOUR POST-DIGESTIVE EFFECT is usually the result of sour taste. It decreases Vata but increases Pitta and Kapha. Like sweet post-digestive effect, it aids in the smooth elimination of feces and urine, but it decreases the reproductive fluid.
- PUNGENT POST-DIGESTIVE EFFECT is usually the result of pungent, bitter and astringent tastes. It decreases Kapha but increases Vata and Pitta. It obstructs the elimination of feces and urine, and diminishes the reproductive fluid.

3. ENERGY OF HERBS – VIRYA

The main energy of herbs is their heating or cooling capacity, which is their most powerful and immediate effect upon our bodily functioning. Called Virya in Sanskrit, it literally means "vigor". Hence, herbs devoid of Virya will be inactive or unable to accomplish anything. Ayurveda speaks of the energy of substances as primarily heating or cooling, recognizing within this classification differences of degrees of hot or cold.

Generally, energy follows taste. Sweet, bitter and astringent tastes are cooling, while salty, sour and pungent tastes are heating. Sweet post-digestive effect is generally cooling in energy, while sour and pungent post-digestive effects are usually heating. Heating or cooling energy generally dominates over taste and post-digestive action as it is stronger and more immediate in its results.

TYPE	ACTION ON DOSHAS	GENERAL EFFECT
Hot	Pacifies Kapha and Vata, Aggravates Pitta	Helps digestion, causes hot sensation, thirst and sweating
Cold	Pacifies Pitta, Aggravates Kapha and Vata	Cooling, exhilarant, moistening, enlivening, increases the tissues

4. Special Potency — Prabhava

Apart from their energetics, herbs possess other special healing properties owing to various reasons. This special or specific potency of an herb is called *Prabhava*. It can be observed that two herbs of similar taste, energy and post-digestive effect differ in action. Although it is difficult to explain the exact nature of Prabhava, it can be due to specific elemental combinations or to specificity in the site of an herb's action (for example, the cardiotonic activity of the herb arjuna).

Types of Prabhava and Examples:

ANTI-TOXIC – Shirisha, plantain

BACTERICIDAL – Guggul, myrrh, garlic

PURGATIVES – Aloe, rhubarb root, senna

GHEE AND MILK – Both are sweet in taste and post-digestive effect and cold in energy but ghee increases Agni while milk does not.

Therapeutic Effects of Herbs

Based upon their energetics, herbs have various therapeutic effects like diaphoretic action (promoting sweating) or diuretic action (increasing urination). This therapeutic effect of herbs is called karma in Sanskrit, which means action. It refers to the action of an herb on the doshas, tissues, waste-materials, systems and organs of the body. All medicinal substances, deriving from the five elements, are first converted into five elemental forms within the body. Then they can influence the respective doshas and systems. This action may be localized, affecting one part of the body, or systemic, affecting the body as a whole. It can be direct, acting through a particular substance within the herb, or indirect, deriving from the process of digestion.

Classification of Herbal Actions

Ayurveda has an entire science of classifying herbal actions so that we can employ herbs in the best possible manner.

Classification By Therapies

Ayurveda classifies healing therapies under two broad categories: Shodhana or purification, and shamana or palliation. Shodhana eliminates the doshas that cause disease, while shamana gradually reduces them. These factors are explained in detail in the next chapter on Ayurvedic therapies.

PURIFICATION (Shodhana) is of five types, which constitutes Pancha Karma or the five purification measures:

1. Emesis (Vamana)
2. Purgation (Virechana)
3. Blood purification (Raktamokshana)
4. Oil-containing enema (Anuvasana)
5. Decoction enema (Asthapana)

PALLIATION THERAPY (Shamana) is of two types: Either building (Brimhana) or reducing (Langhana).

Building (Brimhana) includes oleation (Snehana) and astringent action (Stambhana).

Reducing (Langhana) includes drying (Rukshana) and sudation (Swedana).

Classification By Doshas, Tissues, and Waste-Materials

Therapies can be classified according to their effect on the doshas, tissues and waste-materials which is a direct extension of their energetics. Ayurveda explains the effects of herbs on each of these. Below we provide some prime examples.

Action on Doshas

Vata-reducing	Sesame oil	Vata-aggravating	Beans
Pitta-reducing	Ghee	Pitta-aggravating	Mustard
Kapha-reducing	Honey	Kapha-aggravating	Cheese

Action on Tissues

Increasing plasma (rasa)	Shatavari, amalaki
Blood-cleansing	Turmeric, red clover
Muscle-relaxing	Valerian, jatamamsi
Fat-reducing	Guggul, myrrh
Nourishing bones	Triphala, red coral
Nourishing nerves	Brahmi, shankha pushpi
Increasing reproductive tissue	Ashwagandha, kapikacchu

Action on Waste-materials

Increasing the stool	Barley, psyllium
Promoting sweat	Ginger, cinnamon, basil
Promoting urination	Punarnava, gokshura, uva ursi

Classification by Channel Systems Affected:

Digestive System

Improving taste (Rochana)	Lemon, lime, salt
Digestive stimulants (Dipana)	Asafoetida, fennel
Digestive agents (Pachana)	Dry Ginger, cayenne
Gastric irritant (Vidahi)	Chili
Astringent (Vishtambhi)	Jack fruit, persimmons
Emetic (Vamana)	Emetic nut, lobelia
Anti-emetic (Chardi Nigraha)	Cardamom, fennel

Excretory System

Purgative (Virechana)	Castor oil, trivrit
Anti-diarrhea	Kutaj, alum
Asthapana (corrective enemas)	Dashamula
Anuvasana (medicated oil enemas)	Sesame oil
Anthelmintic (Krimighna)	Vidanga, pumpkin seeds

Respiratory System

Anti-cough (Kasahara)	Sumach, horehound
Anti-asthma (Shwasahara)	Vasa, mullein

Circulatory System

Heart tonic (Hridya)	Arjuna, hawthorne berries
Alterative (Rakta Prasadana	Turmeric, red clover

Urinary System

Promotes urination (Mutrala)	Punarnava, gokshura

Sebaceous System

Promote sweating (Swedana)	Ginger, bayberry

Menstrual System

Promotes menstruation	Turmeric, saffron

Medium of Intake

The effect of herbs also varies according to the medium that we take them with. This is called *Anupana* in Sanskrit. The simplest mediums of intake are hot and cold water but certain foods like milk, spicy herbs that aid in absorption like ginger, and oils like ghee also function in this way. Generally, all herbs for improving digestion are taken with warm, not cold, water in order to facilitate the digestive fire. Milk is also usually taken warm. Anupanas direct the herbs in different ways. Milk brings out their nutritive properties, for example, while honey increases their expectorant action.

Anupanas

Vata	Hot water, ginger tea, warm milk, sesame oil
Pitta	Cool water, warm milk, aloe gel, ghee, butter
Kapha	Hot water, ginger tea, honey, guggul

Dosage of Medicines

The right effect of herbs depends on correct dosage. Excess doses can cause side effects, while doses too small will not be powerful enough to accomplish their aim. Dosage of medicines varies according to constitution, digestive power, strength of the individual, age, disease power, potency of the medicine and condition of the gastrointestinal tract.

The Ayurvedic physician Sharangdhara has suggested that for a one- month old child the dose should be 125 mg. (one Ratti). This amount should be increased at the rate of one Ratti per month, up to one year, when the total will be twelve Rattis or about 1.5 grams. The following approximate doses should be used according to different preparations:

HERBAL PREPARATION	DOSAGE
Expressed juice of herbs (Swarasa), Herbal wines (Asava or Arishtha)	20 ml. (1/2 Pala)
Decoction (Hima, Phanta)	40 ml. (1 Pala)
Powder (Churna)	1- 4 gms. (1/2 Karsha)
Medicated Oils, Ghees, and Herbal Jellies (Taila, Ghrita, Avaleha)	10 gms. (1 karsha)

For Rasayana or rejuvenation therapy, a special type of dosage method is suggested. The dosage of the medicine is gradually increased and then gradually decreased in the same manner, as explained in the section on Vardhamana Rasayana.

Times To Take Medicines (Bhaishajya Kala)

Herbs have different effects relative to the different times at which we take them. To get the best results for a particular condition, herbs should be taken at the appropriate time. In Ayurveda herbs are taken at different times according to factors like daily variations of the doshas, organ reflexes, the state of Agni (the digestive fire), and the stages of digestion:

• ON AN EMPTY STOMACH (Abhakta) —The potency of the herb exerts the strongest action during this time. For strong persons and acute disorders, medicines should be given at this time.

• BEFORE MEALS (Pragbhakta) — For treating obesity, problems of the lower abdomen (Apana Vayu), and toning up the intestinal muscles, medicines should be given at this time.

• DURING THE MEAL (Madhyabhakta) — For disorders of the midabdomen (Samana Vayu), or the digestive nerves, this is the best time.

• AFTER MEALS (Adhobhakta) — For treating the upper abdomen and chest (Vyana and Udana), medicines should be given after meals. This time is also used to treat the diseases above the neck region which are due to excess Kapha.

- MIXED WITH FOOD (Samabhakta) — To suppress the bad taste of medicines and for children and delicate persons, this is the best way to administer herbs. This time is used for persons having an aversion to medicines, or anorexia, and for treating diseases which have spread throughout the entire body.
- BETWEEN LUNCH AND DINNER (Antarabhakta) — This time is best for treating disorders of Vyana Vayu, the outward moving air that governs the circulatory system.
- BOTH BEFORE AND AFTER EATING (Samudga) — For treating diseases like hiccups, trembling, convulsions, and disorders of the lower part of the body, medicines should be given both immediately before and after meals.
- REPEATEDLY (Muhurmuhu) — For treating disorders like cough, hiccup, dyspnea, vomiting and poisoning, medicines should be given repeatedly as long as required.
- WITH EACH MORSEL OF FOOD (Sagrasa) — For stimulating digestion and for taking aphrodisiacs, medicines should be mixed while eating each bite of food.
- BETWEEN BITES OF FOOD (Grasantara) — For treating disorders of the respiratory system (Prana Vayu) this is useful.
- AT NIGHT (Nisha) — For treating diseases of the head, neck, eye, ear, nose and throat, medicines should be given at night.

Routes of Administration

The effect of herbs varies according to their routes of administration or the sites on the body from which we introduce them. The Ayurvedic rule is to treat a condition both systemically, through the body as a whole, and locally, nearest to the site of the disease as possible. Medicines are given primarily through the mouth. After digestion and absorption, they are circulated through the lymph and blood to the rest of the body. But to achieve specific local actions other routes are used. Generally, these work to bring the herbs to a more specific part of the body, like eye applications for eye diseases. However, application to the skin in particular also affects the body as a whole. Enemas are used to bring nourishing substances like oils into the body when the digestion is too weak to absorb them.

Routes of Administration for Medicines

Nose	Medicated nasal drops or powders
Eye	Eye ointments and herbal applications
Ear	For treating diseases of the ear, herbs and oils may be applied at this site
Anus	Enemas
Urethra	Enema is given by this route to treat urinary infections
Vagina	In vaginal and uterine disorders, as suppositories, swabs and douches
Skin	To treat various skin diseases external applications like washes, poultices, plasters and oils

Collection of Herbs

The effects of herbs vary according to when and how we collect them. Since most herbs are purchased commercially, we usually have no way of knowing this except by the reputation of the company. For this reason, we should strive to use organically grown herbs that are as fresh as possible and which have not been kept in storage too long. If we are able to collect our own herbs, we should collect them at a time in which their potency is ready and during a favorable moment.

One should arise before sunrise on an auspicious day. Mondays or Thursdays, the days ruled by the Moon or Jupiter, are particularly good, especially when the Moon is waxing. Wednesday, ruled by Mercury, is also fine. Good signs (as calculated according to Vedic Astrology) for picking herbs for the Moon are Taurus, Cancer, Virgo, Libra and Pisces. Good Nakshatras (lunar constellations) for the Moon are Rohini, Mrigshira, Punarvasu, Pushya, Uttara Phalguni, Hasta, Chitra, Swati, Anuradha, Mula (for roots), Uttarshadha, Shravana, Uttara Bhadra and Revati.

The best time for picking most plants is in the morning. After praying to the Sun and Moon, a special prayer should be done before the particular herb, plant or tree whose part will be taken, seeking the blessings of the herb and access to its healing powers. Then while preserving silence, the plant should be collected. An exception is plants near water, rivers, or lakes. These plants are most potent at night and so should be collected at that time instead.

In India, most herbs become potent between the months of October to December, after the rainy season, which is the main period of collection. In North America and other temperate regions, roots become potent in the fall, leaves and leafy herbs become potent in the spring, and flowers are best just before they open. Individual species have special requirements based upon their active ingredients that should be studied carefully.

An exception to the general rule is collection of medicines for diarrhea, dysentery, and vomiting. These medicines have a drying nature and should be collected in the months of May and June when the weather in India is hot and dry. In temperate regions, such dry weather usually prevails in late summer. In addition, the bark or roots of trees should be cut from the north direction to ensure their greatest energy.

HERBAL CLASSIFICATIONS

Ayurveda describes forty-one prime attributes, through which we can understand the effects of medicines. These come in four groups:

- The twenty qualities of substances (Gurvadi Guna)
- The ten qualities of application (Paradi Guna)

- The five special qualities (Vishishtha Guna)
- The six psychological qualities (Adhyatmika Guna)

The term guna means quality, mode or property. Out of these, only the twenty attributes are used in pharmacology. These twenty properties occur in two groups of ten, as qualities essential for tissue gain or those responsible for tissue loss. The factors which promote new cellular units are termed Samanya or homologous. The factors which promote destruction of tissues are called Vishesha or heterologous.

The Twenty Attributes (Gurvadi Guna)

These are referred to as bodily properties (Sharira Gunas) as they are found in body tissue as well as in the substances which influence them. They are physical as well as pharmacological in action. See Qualities of Food for more information on these attributes.

Twenty Attributes and Their Actions

Guna	Composition	Action
1. Heavy (Guru)	Earth, Water	Building (Brimhana)
2. Light (Laghu)	Fire, Air, Ether	Reducing (Langhana)
3. Cold (Shita)	Water	Cooling (Stambhana)
4. Hot (Ushna)	Fire	Heating (Swedana)
5. Wet (Snigdha)	Water	Moistening (Kledana)
6. Dry (Ruksha)	Earth, Fire, Air	Absorbing (Shoshana)
7. Dull (Manda)	Earth, Water	Slowing-Pacifying (Shamana)
8. Sharp (Tikshna)	Fire	Penetrating-Purifying (Shodhana)
9. Firm (Sthira)	Earth	Stabilizing (Dharana)

Twenty Attributes and Their Actions (cont'd)

Guna	Composition	Action
10. Mobile (Sara)	Air	Stimulating (Prerana)
11. Smooth (Mridu)	Water	Loosening (Shlathana)
12. Hard (Kathina)	Earth	Hardening (Dridhikarana)
13. Clear (Vishada)	Fire, Air, Ether	Cleansing (Kshalana)
14. Sticky (Picchhila)	Earth, Water	Adhering (Lepana)
15. Soft (Shalkshna)	Earth, Water	Healing (Ropana)
16. Rough (Khara)	Air	Scraping (Lekhana)
17. Subtle (Sukshma)	Air, Ether	Pervading (Vivarana)
18. Gross (Sthula)	Earth	Covering (Samvarana)
19. Dense (Sandra)	Earth, Water	Solidifying (Prasadana)
20. Fluid (Drava)	Water	Liquefying (Vilodana)

The Ten Qualities of Application (Paradi Gunas)

These are widely used in treatment and indicate the factors for the right applications of medicines.

1. Para	Preferable, superior grade
2. Apara	Not preferable, inferior grade
3. Yukti	Rationale, method of using
4. Samkhya	Enumeration
5. Samyoga	Combination with other medicines or foods
6. Vibhaga	Division
7. Prithaktva	Separateness

8. Parimana	Proper weights and measures for usages
9. Samskara	Processing to facilitate properties
10. Abhyasa	Repeated use

Ayurvedic practitioners consider various technical factors in prescribing herbs. These include whether the medicines are of superior or inferior quality, whether their inherent power is strong or weak. They must understand the rationale or strategy behind their usage, whether it aims at purification or palliation. They must understand how to use them – the number of their applications, whether they are combined with other substances or divided up into smaller parts, whether they are employed separately or together, in what amount, according to what processing, and in what frequency.

The Five Special Qualities (Vishishtha Gunas)

We must consider the effects of herbs upon the senses and the sensory qualities that they convey directly or indirectly. The five qualities of the senses must be considered:

• Sound, touch, sight, taste and smell (shabda, sparsha, rupa, rasa, gandha)

These are called the five Tanmatras and underlie all perceptible phenomena in the universe. We must consider the impressions (tanmatras) we are receiving in all of our activities in life, including those we gain during treatment or from taking medicines. These can enhance or counteract the effect of treatment.

The Six Psychological Qualities (Adhyatmika Gunas)

We must consider the effects of medicines upon the mind as well as the emotions of the person being treated. The prime mental qualities are:

1) Buddhi, intellect or judgment	2) Iccha, desire
3) Dwesha, aversion	4) Sukha, pleasure
5) Duhkha, pain	6) Prayatna, effort or volition

Each mental state involves these considerations. First we must ascertain (Buddhi) the nature of something. We must determine what it is and what value it may have for us. This leads to attraction (Iccha) to what we have decided is good or wholesome and to repulsion (Dwesha) to what we think is bad or unwholesome. Getting what we think is good gives rise to pleasure (Sukha), while experiencing what we think is bad causes pain (Duhkha). This gives rise to effort or action (Prayatna) to hold on to what gives us happiness and to avoid what causes suffering.

According to Ayurveda, we should seek out those things that provide enduring happiness as opposed to merely following those which yield temporary pleasure. Hence, it is important that we learn to ascertain the inner truth of things. This right judgment is the basis of right effort. No one wants pain, but wrongly seeking lasting happiness in temporary pleasure, the mind gets confused and the result is suffering and disease.

In treatment we must consider the psychological qualities of the patient and how to guide them to right judgment and from that to right action. This is important in Ayurveda, which aims at teaching the patient how to live rightly. The Ayurvedic doctor must also be able to judge the nature of a condition in order to determine the right action to alleviate pain.

THE FIFTY THERAPEUTIC ACTIONS

Charaka has defined fifty groups of herbs according to their therapeutic action. Each group, containing ten herbs, is called a "Mahakashaya." By taking common characteristics into account, other similar herbs can be incorporated into these groups. These groups are as follows:

1. Vitalizing Agents (Jivaniya)	Help protect one's life and promote longevity	Licorice, sesame seeds or mung beans
2. Bulk-Promoting Agents (Brimhaniya)	Increase bodily weight and promote formation of new tissues	Ashwagandha, bala, shatavari, and marshmallow
3. Reducing Agents (Lekhaniya)	Reduce fat or other accumulations	Cyperus, turmeric, black pepper, or barberry
4. Accumulation-Breaking Agents (Bhedaniya)	Break down stronger accumulations like gall stones or kidney stones	Chitrak, kutaj, pashana bheda
5. Healing Agents (Sandhaniya)	Promote the healing of wounds or cuts	Guggul, manjishta, turmeric, aloe gel, bayberry
6. Digestive Stimulants (Dipaniya)	Enkindle the digestive fire (Agni)	Dry ginger, black pepper, long pepper, chitrak, cinnamon, cardamom
7. Tonics (Balya)	Strength-giving herbs	Bala, ashwagandha, shatavari, ginseng
8. Complexion-Improving Agents (Varnya)	Improve skin tone and luster	Sandalwood, turmeric, lotus root, manjishtha
9. Beneficial for the Throat (Kanthya)	For soothing sore throat and improving the voice	Raisins, vidari, bayberry, haritaki, licorice
10. Heart Tonics (Hridya)	Strengthen heart function	Pomegranate fruit, arjuna, mango, hawthorne berries
11. Anti-Saturative (Triptighna)	Relieve false sense of contentment, as under excess Kapha	Calamus, guduchi, ginger
12. Anti-Hemorrhoidal (Arsoghna)	Help heal hemorrhoids	Kutaj, ginger, haritaki, calamus

13. Anti-Dermatitis (Kusthaghna)	Reduce skin inflammations	Catechu, turmeric, haritaki, amalaki, plantain
14. Anti-Pruritic (Kandughna)	Relieve itching on the skin	Neem bark, barberry, licorice
15. Anthelmintic (Krimighna)	Destroy parasites	Vidanga, betel nuts, pumpkin seeds
16. Anti-Toxin (Vishaghna)	Counter poisons	Shirisha, turmeric, licorice, sandalwood
17. Lactogogues (Stanya-Janana)	Promote secretion of breast milk	Shatavari, fennel, dill
18. Lactodepurants (Stanya-Shodhana)	Purify breast milk	Guduchi, ginger, dandelion
19. Spermogenic (Shukra-Janana),	Increase sperm count	Vidari, ashwagandha, shatavari, lotus seeds
20. Purify Sperm (Shukra-Shodhana)	Remove toxins from the sperm	Kushta, bayberry, vetivert
21. Oleating Adjunctive (Snehopaga)	Facilitate absorption of oils	Raisins, licorice, vidari
22. Adjuncts To Sweating Therapy (Swedopaga)	Allow for easier sweating (not diaphoretics or sweat-inducing however)	Castor root, barley, sesame, black gram, mung beans
23. Adjuncts To Emesis (Vamanopaga)	Aid in the process of vomiting	Honey, licorice
24. Adjuncts To Purgation (Virecanopaga)	Usually laxative in nature	Raisins, prunes, haritaki, amalaki
25. Adjuncts To Decoction Enemas (Asthapanopaga)	Cleanse Vata from the colon	Bilwa, pippali, calamus, licorice
26. Adjunctives To Oily Enemas (Anuvasanopaga)	Calm Vata in the colon	Fennel, gokshura, bilwa

27. Adjunctives To Cleansing Nasal Therapy (Shirovire-canopaga)	Remove Kapha from above the neck	Black pepper, long pepper, mustard
28. Anti-Emetics (Chardini-Nigrahana)	Stop vomiting	Cardamom, fresh ginger, vetivert, puffed rice
29. Thirst-Relieving (Trishna-Nigrahana)	Aid in hydration of tissues	Lemon, lime, sandalwood, coriander, ginger (for thirst owing to Kapha)
30. Stop Hiccups (Hikka-Nigrahana)	Relieves hiccup and eructation	Elecampane, haritaki, long pepper
31. Give Form To The Feces (Purisha-Samgraniya)	Astringent and anti-diarrhea	Lodhra, pomegranate husks, some forms of clay
32. Give Color To The Stool (Purisha-Virajiniya)	Improve stool formation	Catechu, lotus root, licorice, sesame seed
33. Anti-Diuretics (Mutra-Sangrahniya)	Stop excessive urination	Bhallataka, rose hips
34. Give Color To The Urine (Mutra-Virajinya)	Improve urine formation	Lotus seed, lotus root, licorice
35. Diuretics (Mutra-Virecaniya)	Promote urinary flow	Gokshura, punarnava, coriander, lemon grass
36. Stop Cough (Kasa-hara)	Anti-tussive	Phyllanthus, haritaki, vasa, raisins, sumach
37. Counter Asthma (Shwasahara)	Stop wheezing, ease breathing	Elecampane, cardamom, basil, ma huang
38. Relieve Edema and Swelling (Shotahara)	Diuretics and astringents	Bilwa and gokshura

39. Febrifuge (Jwara-hara)	Relieve fevers	Draksha, manjishta, tulsi, raw sugar, bitters generally
40. Relieve Fatigue (Shramahara)	As from overexposure to heat	Dates, pomegranate juice, sugar cane, raisins
41. Relieve Burning Sensation On The Skin Daha-Prasha-mana)	Anti-inflammatory	Sandalwood, vetivert, lotus leaf, raw sugar
42. Relieve Cold Sensation On The Skin Shita-Prashamana)	Stimulate circulation on the skin	Valerian, agaru, calamus, long pepper, ginger, coriander
43. Relieve Skin Rashes (Udarda-Prashamana)	As for urticaria	Catechu, arjuna
44. Relieve Body Ache (Angamarda-Prashama)	Cure malaise, as from fever or flu	Sandalwood, cardamom, mint, camphor
45. Relieve Colic Pain (Shula-Prashamana)	Analgesic and anti-spasmodic for smooth muscle	Fennel, dill, asafoetida, cardamom, ginger, long pepper
46. Stopping Bleeding (Shonita-Sthapana)	Hemostatic	Licorice, lodhra, honey, red clay, agrimony
47. Relieve Pain (Vedana-Sthapana)	Sedatives for nerve pain	Valerian, jatamamsi, shirisha, bayberry
48. Restore Consciousness (Samja-Stapana)	As from coma or delirium	Gotu kola (brahmi), calamus, asafoetida, camphor
49. Promote Reproduction (Praja-Sthapana)	Cure sterility, remove obstructions in genital tract	Amalaki, haritaki, gotu kola (brahmi), katuka
50. Promote Longevity (Vaya-Sthapana)	Rejuvenative, counter the aging process	Guduchi sattva, haritaki, gotu kola, shatavari, amalaki

COMMON GROUPS OF HERBS

The following herbal formulas are commonly used in Ayurveda either by themselves or as part of greater formulas. They provide the reader with a good idea of the herbal preparations typical to Ayurveda.

Triphala, the three fruits	Haritaki, bibhitaki, amalaki	For all doshas, particularly for Vata	Laxative, alter-ative, anti-arthrit-ic, calm-ative, rejuvenative
Trikatu, the three spices	Dry ginger, long pep-per, black pepper	Reduces Ama and Kapha, increases Agni	Stimulant, diges-tive, expectorant
Trijata	Cinnamon, carda-mom, cinnamon leaf	Reduces Ama and stimulates Prana and Agni	Carminative, anti-spasmodic, aro-matic, anti-emetic
Chaturjata	Trijata and nagake-shar	Reduces Ama, stimulates Agni and circulation	Carminative, stimulant, ap-petizer
Trimada	Vidanga, cyperus, chitrak	Clears conscious-ness, opens chan-nels, removes obstructions	Stimulant, deob-struent
Chaturbija, the four seeds	Fenugreek, water-cress, kalajaji, yavani	Promotes move-ment of water and energy	Carminative, stimulant, diuretic
Panchakola	Long pepper (pip-pali), pippali root, chavya, chitrak, dry ginger	Increases Agni and burns Ama	Digestive, stimu-lant
Panchaval-kala the five barks	Barks of nyagrodha, udumbara, ash-wat-tha, plaksha, parisha	Promotes healing after injury or infection, mainly anti-Pitta	Astringent, styp-tic, anti-diuretic, hemostatic

Panchapallava	Mango, jambu, kapittha, citron, bilwa	for diabetes, poor absorption, intestinal inflammation	Astringent, stomachic anti-diarrhea
Trinapancha Mula	Kusha, kasa, nala, darbha, sugar cane	Eases urination, counters urinary infections	Diuretic, alterative, for urinary tract stones
Panchatikta, the five bitters	Vasa, guduchi, neem, kantakari, patola	For fever, convalescence and weak digestion	Antipyretic, febrifuge, alterative, expectorant
Brihat Panchamula, the greater five roots	Bilwa, patala, agnimantha, syonaka, sambhari	Specially alleviates Vata	Diuretic, tonic, antirheumatic
Laghu Panchamula, The lesser five roots	Shalaparni, prishniparni, kantakari, gokshura, brihati	Specially alleviates Vata	Diuretic, tonic, antirheumatic
Dashamula, the ten roots	Combines Brihat and Laghu Panchamula	Specially alleviates Vata	Antirheumatic, analgesic, good for basti enema therapy)

Combinations with Ashwagandha

Ashwagandha is the prime tonic used in Ayurveda, with a position in the Ayurvedic materia medica similar to that of ginseng in Chinese medicine (the two plants, however, are not botanically related). Combined with different herbs, it becomes an excellent tonic for various organs and systems of the body.

Ashwagandha Combinations

Ashwagandha and shatavari	Tonic for reproductive system (male or female)
Ashwagandha and gotu kola (or Brahmi)	Tonic for brain and nerves
Ashwagandha and arjuna	Tonic for heart
Ashwagandha and vidari kanda	Tonic for bones; anti-arthritic
Ashwagandha and gokshura	Tonic for kidneys and bladder
Ashwagandha and bala	Tonic for lungs and muscles
Ashwagandha and kapikacchu	Excellent aphrodisiac

Combinations with Aloe Vera

Aloe is an excellent herb that combines both tonifying and reducing actions, having both a cleansing and building effect. It also can serve as a medium in which to take other herbs and enhances their potency.

Aloe Combinations

Aloe and turmeric	Cleanses liver and blood, promotes menstruation, aids in healing of wounds
Aloe and ginger	Stimulates digestion, removes mucus
Aloe and licorice	Antacid, demulcent, protects mucus membranes
Aloe and gentian	Bitter tonic
Aloe and golden seal	Natural anti-biotic
Aloe and saffron	Female reproductive system tonic

PHARMACEUTICAL ASPECTS OF AYURVEDA

It is not enough to have the right herbs to treat a condition, one must use them in the right preparation. The herbs must be in a form in which their potency is enhanced and preserved. The knowledge of how to prepare medicines is called "pharmaceutics". Correct knowledge of this is an important part of Ayurveda.

Ayurveda contains a vast pharmaceutical science for preparing pills, powders, herbal extracts, herbal wines, medicated oils and ghees, and herbal confections, as well as many special mineral preparations. Many companies in India today prepare hundreds of such Ayurvedic medicines both for doctors and for over the counter use. Ayurvedic herb and medicine stores can be found throughout the country. They require no prescription to buy or to use.

Ayurvedic medicines are divided into three classes, according to their material of origin:

• Herbal

• Mineral

• Animal

While considering herbal medicines, many factors are important beginning with the part of the plant that is best for usage: The root, flower, stem, leaves, bark, or exudations like the resin. Similarly, the proper season for collection is noted and signs that the plant is ready for harvesting.

While using mineral substances, the place where the minerals are found, their qualities like color, smell, and form, and their different varieties are important. In the case of animal substances, the creature's habitat, age, sex, food habits, and the part of the animal used should be properly studied.

Properties of the medicine like taste, energy, post-digestive effect, specific action, and various qualities must be taken into account. The action of the medicine on the particular dosha, organ or disease condition in the body to be treated must be considered. While preparing a medicine, a physician must know whether the substance is pure or impure – whether it can be used directly or if it requires special processes to remove its side effects and enhance its benefits. If it is impure, the methods of its purification must be known. If a particular substance is not available at a particular season, appropriate substitutes should be known.

List of Ayurvedic Preparations

Ayurveda employs an entire range of herbal preparations from the raw plant to complex pharmaceutical products.

- Kwatha, Decoction
- Phanta, Hot infusion
- Hima, Cold infusion
- Swarasa, Fresh juice
- Kalka, Crushed pulp of the plant
- Ghana, Decoction evaporated to solid
- Arka, Liquid extracts
- Avaleha, Herbal jellies
- Asava and Arista, Herbal wines or tinctures
- Churna, Powders
- Ghrita, Medicated ghee
- Kshara, Extraction of alkalis from plants
- Lavana, Salts
- Guggul, Resins and balsams
- Lepa, Pastes
- Upanaha, Poultices
- Malahara, Ointments
- Panak, Crushed fruit and their preparations
- Sattva, Active or concentrated herb principles and extracts
- Taila, Medicated oils
- Varti, Suppositories
- Guti-vati, Tablets
- Bhasma, Oxide ashes
- Sara, Resins

- Kshira, Exudations, like the milky juice from various tropical fig trees
- Anjana, Ointments
- Dravaka, mixture of ashes of plants, salts, and alkalies distilled to produce a liquid, like Shankhadrava
- Druti, Solid substances converted into liquids, like liquefied sulphur

Purification of Medicines

Many herbs and minerals require special purification processes in order for their beneficial properties to be usable and their side effects removed. For purification of herbs, many methods exist including to cleanse, sort, peel, unhusk, polish, strain, filter, distill, or dehydrate the substance. For purification of metals and minerals, complicated and time-consuming processes are necessary like trituration, boiling in milk or cow's urine, soaking in vinegar, or keeping the substance for a long time in dairy products like buttermilk.

The modern medical pharmaceutical industry requires a range of various chemicals or solvents in its preparations. The Ayurvedic pharmaceutical industry, on the other hand, uses the contact of minerals with heat along with certain purifying herbal substances or juices. The simplest procedure for preparation of medicines in Ayurveda consists of crushing the leaves and taking out the juice of the herb. Complex procedures may involve sequential processes spread over a period of up to thirty years, like the preparation of Abhrak Bhasma (oxide of mica).

Ayurveda does not use heavy metals or minerals without extensive processes to render them fit for human consumption. In this regard, it uses drugs medicinally but in a careful, complex and safe manner. Mercury or gold preparations (rasas), for example, require many physical and subtle chemical processes before their final stage is achieved and they are able to be consumed. Such Ayurvedic drugs do not accumulate in the tissues but are eliminated from the body once their work is done. In this way, Ayurveda can employ the great healing power of minerals while avoiding their side effects. Ayurvedic medicines thus are much more complex than simple herbal or drug preparations. They have an efficacy greater than either, while preserving the benefits of both.

The most important factor in the preparation of an Ayurvedic medicine is Agni, or heat, which transforms the substance so that it can be accepted by the human body and become easily absorbed. Agni is important for bringing about the transformation of qualities required in various pharmaceutical processes. With the help of heat or Agni, many processes like heating, frying, melting, burning, smoking, cleansing, drying, distillation, digestion and oxidation are carried out.

During ancient times, although there was no equipment to measure heat gradations, various grades of heat were specifically described like low, medium, high, very high and extremely high. For these, certain parameters were used like the temperature at which hay burns, at which ammonium chloride melts, or at which borax crystallizes. For controlling temperature at various levels, different heating methods were used like sand bath, water bath, oil bath and sulphur-melting bath. These are still in use today. Various qualities of heat were obtained from different sources like cow dung, sheep dung, horse dung, woods like catechu, coal of different woods, and the husks of rice.

Purification Procedures

Ayurveda uses elaborate purification procedures to make toxic substances safe for internal usage. Procedures like trituration, contact heating, closed-shell heating, and heating in boiling liquid sulphur also indicate the portion of the body in which the medicine's action is likely to take place.

In *Khalvi* preparations, minerals are triturated with liquid extracts of herbs. A powder of the mineral is placed into a mortar and pestle with the juice of an herb and it is triturated (stirred in a clockwise motion with the pestle) until completely dry. This is one *Bhavana* or procedure. Bhavanas are done at least seven times but, in some instances, may occur over a thousand times. Such medicines act mainly on the upper part of the gastrointestinal tract, because the heat applied in this process is nothing but friction between mortar and pestle during trituration. This process of trituration is also the basis for the other preparations that follow.

In *Parpati* preparations, first Kajjali or "humanized" Rasa (sulphur and mercury) is prepared. Other herbs and minerals are then added one by one and triturated to create Kajjali powder. The components are next heated on an iron plate, which is just hot enough to liquefy the combination. Then the mixture is taken out and put on a banana leaf and allowed to cool. As this process requires more heat than the Khalvi group, these medicines do not break down as quickly. They dissolve in the middle portion of the gastrointestinal tract and therefore act on the small intestine. Hence, medicines to improve absorption are prepared in this manner.

Still further micro-refined products materialize in the process of preparing the *Kupipakva* group. Kajjali is taken, along with certain medicines triturated in it, put into a glass shell and fired together usually in sand for a period of twenty-four to seventy-two hours. This produces Rasa or alchemical preparations using Kajjali or humanized mercury-sulphur as a base. Here the heat contact is such that the ingredients must be put into a closed glass shell. The heat applied is much higher than that for the Khalvi group. Two different products result from this process, one at the sublimated portion at the neck of a glass shell or bottle, and the other in the sedimented portion at the bottom.

Even though both these products arise from the same initial ingredients, the substances in the sublimated portion and those in the sedimented portion differ in their elemental constituents. Those found in the neck portion act on the lung, heart, and brain, or upper part of the body, while those at the bottom are more compact and act on pelvic organs like the uterus and kidneys and the lower part of the body.

Kupi prepared medicines are refined further, which produces yet a stronger bond between the medicines (sulphur and mercury). In the *Pottali* group, a sulphur cooking medium is used. The medicines are placed in a cloth bag and immersed in boiling sulphur for up to six hours. Sulphur imparts heat from all sides to the particles of the formula suspended within it. These drugs are meant for quick action, which may be sublingual. Their action is on deeper tissues and works directly through the brain. The best example is Hemagarbha or purified gold.

Preparation of Bhasmas

Oxidation of metals is a specialty of Ayurvedic pharmaceutical processes. The substances resulting from this are called *Bhasmas*, which literally means ashes. These are primarily oxides of the metals but their exact chemical nature requires further scientific analysis.

For hard metals the following procedure is used. Each metallic substance, in the form of a flattened piece, is heated on charcoal and then dipped into sesame oil, buttermilk, cow's urine, kanji (fermented wheat gruel), and a decoction of horsegram. In each of these mediums, the metal is heated and dipped seven times. When it is purified, the metal becomes brittle and another process called Marana is performed. The purified metal is put into an earthen shell on which another earthen shell is made. It is sealed airtight with a cloth dipped in clay. When the shell is dry, it is heated on coals made from the wood of special trees or from cow dung. Heat is applied for six to eight hours and the Bhasma is finished. This procedure may be repeated many times for preparing certain Bhasmas.

Many tests are done to prove that such Bhasmas are ready. These tests differ for different Bhasmas. For example, Copper Bhasma put into lime juice should not turn green. If the Bhasma does not pass the test, it is subjected to repeated firings until it does. Lighter minerals like coral, conch shell and gypsum are heated in the shell for six hours and then they are ready. They require only one heating.

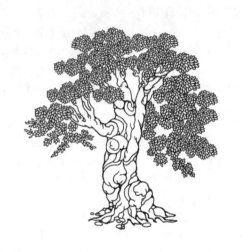

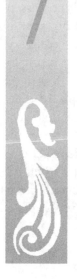

7 The Disease Process According to Ayurveda

> The physician who, though knowing the disease, does not reach the inner self of the patient with the light of his knowledge, will not succeed in his treatment.
> —*Charaka*

CAUSE OF DISEASE

According to Ayurveda, disease is not complicated or mysterious. The causes of health and disease lie in our own every day nature and behavior. In order to treat a disease, we must first understand what has brought it about. We cannot remove an effect without removing its cause. Ayurveda is concerned with going to the root of disease, not merely with treating symptoms. For this it looks at one's entire lifestyle.

According to Ayurveda, the imbalance of the three doshas of Vata, Pitta and Kapha is the immediate cause of all diseases. External factors like weather changes, or internal factors like wrong emotions, can trigger these imbalances. The Ayurvedic view of disease primarily stresses internal causes that can be managed by right living practices and corrected by natural healing methods.

Charaka points out the factors responsible for keeping a person free from disease. He states that one who follows a wholesome diet and life regimen; who enters into actions only after their proper consideration; who is unattached to the pleasures of the senses; whose thought, speech, and deeds are happily blended; whose mind is controlled and is possessed of knowledge, austerity, and the love for meditation; such a person seldom gets afflicted with disease. If we act contrary to these principles, the doshas become aggravated resulting in various health problems.

The three doshas are disturbed by inappropriate diet, behavior and lifestyle. Their imbalance initiates pathological changes such as the build up of toxins. In Ayurveda, the etiology of disease is described in two broad categories: General factors common to all diseases, and specific factors behind particular diseases. A third factor behind disease occurs from the natural effect of time and the aging process. We will explain these factors in detail.

COMMON CAUSES FOR ALL DISEASES

Role of the Senses

One of the most important factors in the disease process is wrong use of the senses. Sight, sound, touch, taste and smell are the five sense qualities through which environmental factors enter the body and mind. How we use our senses determines the type of food that we eat, the water we drink, and the particular lifestyle that we follow.

Sensory contacts are of four types: Excess, deficient, inappropriate and optimal. For example, we can take in too much light through the eyes, too little light, the wrong type of light, or the appropriate type and amount. Out of these four, only optimal contact promotes health. The three other contacts cause disease.

Scientific studies show that disturbing sounds produce pathological changes in the blood. All of us have experienced how noise can disturb not only the mind but also the body. Just as sounds that are too loud can damage health, the same is true of harmful exposure to the other sensory qualities of sight, taste, odor, and touch. An excess of sensations disturbs the mind and leads to wrong actions and dietary indiscretions.

Other medical sciences are beginning to discover this factor in diseases. However, only in Ayurveda are the senses given clear recognition as one of the primary causes of disease. Ayurveda covers not only physical factors but psychological factors as well. The senses are common factors that connect the two. If we look at disease only according to external pathogens and do not acknowledge the role of the senses, we miss much of the real problem. The senses are our real link to the outer world and our relationship with our environment, healthful or unhealthful, can be measured by how we use them. Sensory impressions are like food for the mind and determine how we think, feel and judge things.

Wrong Use of the Will

The second main factor in the disease process is volitional transgression or wrong use of the will. It is called Prajnaparadha, which literally means "failure of intelligence", referring to human weakness by which we continue to perform wrong actions even after we have experienced them to be harmful. An example is an alcoholic who, even after having experienced a hangover and the side effects of drinking, perhaps swearing never to drink again, ignores this message of experience and starts drinking again. Wrong use of the will relates to causes from within our psyche that result in defective, excessive or perverted actions of body, speech and mind.

Unfortunately, most of us today are taught to indulge our senses and to pursue desire rather than to cultivate our will power and enjoy freedom from external influences. Not knowing the proper use of the will, we create many unnecessary problems for ourselves. Ayurveda states that unless we strengthen our will and reduce our desires, we can never have health, much less peace and happiness in life. We will be pulled in various directions by conflicting desires and never experience true happiness and contentment which cannot come through mere external stimulation. To counter this, we must cultivate a strong will and learn to achieve the lasting goals of life: Contentment, creativity and greater awareness.

Misuse of the Body

Maintaining the proper and timely discharge of our natural functions ensures health, while their misuse causes disease. The misuse of bodily functions occurs mainly through either suppression or through forced excitation of our natural urges, what modern psychology calls repression or indulgence. According to Ayurveda, we should not unduly suppress our natural urges but should attend to them attentively as they naturally arise. If we suppress them, we derange and weaken the life-force (Prana) and cause our natural impulses toward healthy function to be impaired. Nor should we artificially excite our urges through the pursuit of self-indulgence. We should seek wholesome sensations and avoid those that are artificial or extreme.

While modern culture has emphasized removing repression, it has not always properly criticized the dangers of over indulgence. A toxic body creates wrong urges that indulgence only reinforces, turning them eventually into addictions that are hard to overcome. The rule is that if we are ever in doubt, repression is safer than indulgence, though a balanced approach is best of all.

Misuse of the Mind

Like the body, the mind has its proper and timely functions that must be maintained for health and well-being. We should train and exercise our mind through regular concentration, contemplation and meditation. Wrong actions of the mind bring about wrong actions of the body and eventually result in disease. The mind gets disturbed owing to an increase in agitated (Rajasic) and dull (Tamasic) qualities in the mind, like wrong imagination or lack of attention. This causes the development of fear, grief, anger, greed, infatuation, envy and other negative emotions which imbalance both the body and the mind. To counter this, we should develop Sattva (clarity, contentment and peace) and avoid distraction and laziness.

Misuse of Speech

Speech is our main organ of action that determines how we function and relate in the world. It has a great power to either help or to harm others. There is perhaps nothing as destructive as harsh words and nothing as helpful as kind and considerate statements. Speech, therefore, has a key place in health and disease.

Misuse of speech refers to using language that is insinuating, untrue, untimely, quarrelsome, unpleasant, incoherent, harsh or abrasive. This not only harms others but also sets up negative energy patterns that harm ourselves as well.

In short, any willful disregard for the natural condition and right usage of things, followed by wrong action or misconduct, is known as volitional transgression. Hence, one should use caution and not indulge in overuse or misuse of any function related to mind, body and speech.

Wrong use of the will and wrong use of the senses usually go together because, without the proper will power, our senses control us rather than us controlling our senses. Two important principles can help in keeping the will and senses directed productively rather than destructively. The first is to hold to non-violence and never wish harm to another living creature in thought, word or deed. The second is detachment, to remain above all desires, fears, enticements and allurements, accepting what life brings us. Then both body and mind will remain calm, centered and relaxed.

Effect of Time

The nature of living beings is to die. What has a beginning must have an end. The effect of time, or the natural movement of change and transformation, is another cause of disease that no one can avoid. No one can escape the effects of seasonal changes and variations governed by the time factor from birth to death. Normal as well as abnormal seasonal changes affect the doshas, the mind and the strength of the body.

Similarly, each individual must face the natural process of aging. Disease naturally occurs through the process of growing old, particularly chronic diseases like arthritis. Although to minimize this certain methods like seasonal regimens and rejuvenation therapies are prescribed, one cannot avoid this altogether, nor should one try. Ayurveda says that we should live a happy life accepting old age when it comes, which has its beauty and wisdom, not trying to be forever young, which is not possible.

Factors Responsible for Aggravation of the Doshas

To prevent disease from arising, we must recognize the factors that cause it - in Ayurvedic terms, recognizing factors that can aggravate the doshas. Physical diseases occur owing to the aggravation of the bodily doshas of Vata, Pitta and Kapha and mental diseases arise from the aggravation of the mental doshas of Rajas and Tamas. Food, drink or environments with similar properties to the doshas cause them to increase and produce disease, for example, drinking cold water which is cold and damp in properties increases Kapha. Behavior of the same nature as the doshas is also responsible for disease, like a Pitta or fiery person spending too much time in the hot sun.

Ayurvedic texts describe in detail the various factors responsible for aggravating Vata, Pitta and Kapha. Disturbed doshas, individually or in combination, damage the tissues and give rise to organic or structural diseases. In the same way, specific causes for a wide of variety of diseases are also described in Ayurveda.

PATHOGENESIS OF DISEASE

Branch and Trunk

According to Ayurveda, the body is divided into three parts: The trunk, the limbs or branches, and the head.

- TRUNK (Koshtha) – Contains the gastro-intestinal tract and most of the organs of the body and has a more hollow space;

- BRANCHES (Shakha) – Or four limbs, which contain primarily solid tissues;
- HEAD-NECK PORTION – Which has a structure that is intermediate containing both solid tissues and hollow organs.

Formation and Appearance of the Doshas

To treat the doshas we must understand their patterns of production, accumulation and movement. The food digested by an individual produces the energy necessary for exercise or for work. The energy so consumed by the body cannot be shown as a weighable or measurable entity. This means that although food builds the tissues that are measurable, some part of it leaves the body in the form of energy that cannot be seen physically.

Every day the doshas appear in the hollow organs of the digestive tract (Koshtha), having moved there from the solid tissues of the branches (Shakha). This happens according to different factors like the stages of digestion, the movement of the doshas through the cycles of time like day and night, and the process of aging. Kapha appears in the chest and upper abdomen, Pitta in the mid-abdomen, and Vata in the lower abdomen. In the digestive process, the doshas appear in the trunk (digestive tract) and after the digestion of food, they again go back to the branches (head and limbs).

The movement of the doshas toward the gastrointestinal tract, or central pull, is their natural flow and helps eliminate their excess states. The force pushing the doshas toward the solid tissues, or peripheral movement, on the other hand, becomes dominant mainly in disease states. It takes the excess doshas from the digestive tract and into the tissues where they cause harm. Once the doshas are deposited in the branches, they mix with the tissues and get stuck there and do not easily come back to the gastrointestinal tract. They remain in the solid tissues and form various diseases according to their nature.

Various factors like excessive exercise, hot weather, too much spicy food and erratic behavior push the doshas toward the branches and cause disease. A person should avoid such factors as soon as one notices the hints of an approaching illness. One should rest, avoid strong stimuli and keep away from entertainment that is likely to be disturbing. In this way, we can prevent the adverse movement of the doshas behind the disease process. Such is the basis of Ayurvedic health recommendations.

Physical and mental rest, avoidance of exciting stimuli, and concentration of the mind on recovery from disease aid in the movement of the doshas back to the gastrointestinal tract. For this, oil and sweating therapies (oleation and sudation) are helpful. Similarly, control of Vata through calming Yoga postures, avoiding sudden contraction or relaxation of the muscles, is another important factor.

PATHOGENESIS OF SPECIFIC DISEASES, THE SIX STAGES OF DISEASE

Our physical bodies are conditioned to certain variations in the environment and to the stresses these create. Only when the stress exceeds our limits does the disease process begin. Ayurveda divides the disease process into six stages or six times for treatment (Shat-Kriyakalas). These stages determine the nature of the therapies required in order to prevent the disease from developing further.

Six Stages of Disease and Treatment

1. ACCUMULATION (Sanchaya)	Of the doshas at their sites in the body
2. PROVOCATION (Prakopa)	Of the doshas when they develop readiness to spread
3. SPREAD (Prasara)	Of the doshas throughout the body

4. RELOCATION (Sthana-sanshraya)	Interaction of the doshas with the tissues (Dhatus) along with their deposit in various parts of the body. In this stage, the initial symptoms of a disease appear
5. MANIFESTATION (Vyakti)	Of the appearance of the characteristic signs and symptoms of the particular disease
6. DIFFERENTIATION (Bheda)	Arising of complications or recovery, ending with cure, disability, or death

The first three stages of accumulation, provocation and spread are part of general or systemic abnormalities of the doshas rather than particular diseases. The next three stages of relocation, manifestation and differentiation relate to the manifestation of the particular disease and the pathological changes occurring in the tissues and organs of the body. The earlier the physician checks the development of the disease, the better the results. The specific signs and symptoms of the aggravated doshas in various stages of accumulation, provocation and spread are clearly described in Ayurvedic texts. The Ayurvedic doctor must identify the stage a particular dosha is passing through so that he can prevent further development of the disease process.

In the relocation phase, the accumulated doshas combine with the damageable factors or bodily tissues (Dushya) and harm them. This is called "the coming together of the disease-causing factors and the sites of disease" (Dosha-Dushya Sammurchhana). The spread of the doshas to the tissues takes place through the channel systems like the blood and lymph vessels, and cellular spaces.

At some level, in the beginning or during the process of pathogenesis, the Agni or digestive power is impaired and a new, unwanted product forms. This toxic accumulation of poor digestion is called "Ama" in Ayurveda. Ama can be produced at any level of digestion and assimilation or at the end stages when body tissues are formed. There are five factors of pathogenesis:

• The aggravated doshas

• The damaged tissues (Dushya) and the interaction of the doshas with these sites that they damage

• The movement of the doshas into the body channels through which nutrient material and waste matter or metabolic by-products normally flow

• Influence on Agni, the digestive juices, enzymes and hormones

• The formation of Ama or impaired and unwanted products of poor digestion and metabolism

It is worth noting here that immunity or resistance to disease is the most important factor for the prevention of a disease or for reducing the severity of an attack. The aim of Ayurveda is to promote health, or the natural state of balance, in order to increase immunity and resistance to disease and to cure disease. A strong immune system prevents the doshas from initiating the disease process.

Knowledge of the disease process is important because it allows us to break or check the spread of the harmful doshas from the beginning - from the stage of accumulation - or before the disease really manifests itself. After the disease is established, such knowledge helps us cure the disease or gain relief before it becomes chronic and its complications start. If the disease is already chronic, this knowledge helps to limit the disability caused or to allow for rehabilitation.

STAGES OF DISEASE AND YOGA PROCEDURES

According to Ayurveda, there are five major factors that usually take part in the pathogenesis of every disease. These are:

• Aggravation of the doshas

• Suppression of the digestive fire (Agnimandya)

- Accumulation of Ama or toxins
- Obstruction in channels (Srotorodha)
- Loss of tissue resistance (Dushya-vaigunya)

Although in the majority of diseases all five factors are involved, diseases do occur which are produced by the predominance of only one of these. A disease like rheumatoid arthritis (Ama-Vata) is produced mainly by Ama, while for indigestion weakness of the digestive power plays the predominant role. In ascites, blockage of the channels is the major factor. Bronchial asthma arises mainly through the aggravation of the doshas. In tuberculosis of the lungs, the loss of tissue resistance is the important factor producing the disease. If, along with routine Ayurvedic treatment, different Yoga procedures are used to remove these pathogenic factors, better and quicker results are obtained. This information should be cross-referenced with descriptions of such Yoga procedures for those who wish to use them in this manner. (Note chapter II. 8 on Yoga and Ayurveda for more information on this).

Weak Digestive Fire

Suppression of the digestive fire, which means defective or low digestive power, plays an important part in many diseases. Many diseases can be improved, if not cured, by increasing the power of Agni or the capacity to convert food properly. For this purpose, Kapalabhati, Suryabhedana and Bhastrika types of Pranayama are useful. Agnisara also helps to increase the digestive capacity.

Ama Formation

Ama is the toxic by-product of indigestion. Formation of Ama takes place because of low digestive power. Ama occurs at two levels in the gastrointestinal tract and at the tissue level. To get rid of these toxins, Vatasara is very useful. Patients should practice Pranayama with inhalation and exhalation done in a one-to-two proportion.

Blockage of the Channels

Often Ama or excess Kapha gets lodged in channels and causes blockage or obstruction resulting in pain and disease. First the patient should be examined properly to ascertain whether Ama is still there. After making certain that the Ama has been removed, yogic purificatory actions are performed accordingly. Pavanamuktasana in particular helps get rid of such obstructions.

Loss of Tissue Resistance

According to different pathologies, different organs, tissues, or systems get damaged and lose their tone and power. When the resistance of the tissues is weakened, we more easily come down with disease. Different yogic procedures can be good for these. For example, for obesity, Dhanurasana (bow pose) and Halasana (plough pose) are useful. For asthma, Jala Neti and Bhastrika are good.

Aggravated Doshas

According to the dominance of the doshas in a particular disease, a specific group of Asanas can be suggested. These are indicated under *Yoga Postures for Different Constitutions*.

8 Ayurvedic Forms of Diagnosis

Ayurveda defines the human being as a combination of the five elements along with the perceiving principle (soul or Atman). The five elements are present in the body in the form of the doshas, tissues and waste-materials comprising the various organs and systems. The soul activates the body from a point beyond it. Between these two is the mind, which coordinates the functions of the soul and the physical body, allowing the soul to work through the body. Thus, the human being has three aspects as physical, mental and spiritual. The period of time during which all these aspects exist and function together is called life.

Body, mind and soul always try to maintain perfect coordination and harmony. Such a condition is known as health. An imbalance in this harmony, even by slight changes in any one of these aspects, makes for ill-health or disease. The duty of the physician is to diagnose the disease and to recommend appropriate measures to correct these disorders. A proper diagnosis forms the basis for proper treatment. There are various methods of patient examination in Ayurveda.

Methods of Clinical Examination

Ayurveda recognizes three means of valid knowledge:

1) Authoritative knowledge (Aptopadesha) received from

179

experienced and authoritative individuals

2) Direct perception (Pratyaksha)

3) Inference (Anumana), the conclusions based upon sound reasoning

1. AUTHORITATIVE KNOWLEDGE

Most of what we learn is passed down in the form of written or spoken teachings from various qualified teachers. Such authoritative knowledge is available in three forms:

• Knowledge from authoritative texts, like Ayurvedic books

• Oral evidence from recognized teachers or authorities who are learned and speak the truth about the matter

• Knowledge about the disease available from the patient and those who know them who have right information about it

The main mode of obtaining information from the patient is by questioning the patient about relevant conditions. This examination by interrogation is an essential part of diagnosis and should be recorded in writing and analyzed carefully. It should include the patient's name; sex; age; place of residence; occupation; location and nature of the disease; onset and duration of the disease; known causes of the disease; symptoms and signs of the disease in respect to sound, touch, sight, taste, and smell; aggravation or alleviation of signs and symptoms; after-effects, complications and sequela; attempts at treatment; and the effect or result of any remedial measures.

Many other factors are useful for the physician to know, about which the patient can provide helpful information. The information so given by the patient or patient history is recorded in the clinical case sheet in a systematic way under the following headings:

• Chief complaint

• History of present illness

• Past medical history

• Family medical history

• Personal, occupational, and social history

2. DIRECT PERCEPTION

The knowledge obtained by the correlation of the soul, mind, sense organs and sense objects is known as direction perception (Pratyaksha). The physician should intelligently apply his senses to examine the patient. The different forms of examination relative to the different senses are as follows:

Examination with the Ear or Auscultation

The intestinal sounds, the sounds of the joints, variations in the voice of the patient or other sounds occurring in any part of the body, including cardiac and respiratory sounds, should be examined with the ear or stethoscope.

Examination with the Eye or Inspection

Much can be seen through an examination of the appearance of the patient, not only through the face but also through the hands and skin. The colors, shapes, proportions and luster, the healthy or diseased look of the body and whatever else that is visible in the body of the patient should be inspected thoroughly with the help of the sense of vision.

For example, high Vata exhibits dull skin tone or dark spots on the skin. High Pitta is evidenced by a reddish tinge to the skin, inflammation or subcutaneous bleeding. High Kapha appears as pallor, puffiness, cysts or fat nodules on the skin.

Examination with the Sense of Taste

The examination of the patient's body by the sense of taste is prohibited and should be done indirectly by inference, or by various laboratory tests.

Examination by the Nose or by Smell

The smell of the doshas, tissues, and waste-materials in the entire body of the patient should be noted as to whether they are normal or abnormal.

Palpation or Examination by Tactile Sense

The normal or abnormal feelings of the patient's tissues and organs can be detected with the help of the tactile sense, by hand. Hot and cold, soft and hard, rough and smooth, and other qualities of the tissues and organs can be used to determine the doshas and tissues affected by the disease.

3. INFERENCE

Inference is reasoning based on sound observations. The state of the digestive fire can be determined by the patient's power of digestion, the patient's strength by the capacity for exercise, the condition of the sense organs by the clarity of perception, and the quality of the mind by the power of concentration. The patient's capacity for understanding is revealed by their goals in life; their emotional state by the strength of their attachments; their infatuation by their lack of understanding; their anger by acts of violence; grief by despondency; joy by exhilaration; pleasure from the sense of satisfaction; fear from dejection; vitality by enthusiasm for undertakings; faith by the opinions they hold; intelligence by their power of reason and recollection; character by their conduct; and aversions by what they refuse to do.

Latent diseases can be revealed by testing with therapeutic or provocative medications. The severity of the disease is revealed by the intensity of the provocative factors, the imminence of death by the fatal prognostic signs, the expectation of recovery by wholesome inclinations, and clarity of mind from the absence of mental perturbation.

TENFOLD EXAMINATION OF PATIENT STRENGTH

For adequate management, it is essential to evaluate the exact strength of the patient as well as the disease. For this, Charaka advocates a tenfold clinical examination (Dashavidha Pariksha).

1. Body constitution (Prakriti)
2. Disease condition (Vikriti)

3. Tissue vitality (Sara)

4. Body build (Samhanana)

5. Body measure (Pramana)

6. Adaptability (Satmya) to food, herbs, and climate

7. Mental constitution (Sattva)

8. Capacity of digestion (Ahara Shakti)

9. Capacity of exercise (Vyayama Shakti)

10. Age (Vayas)

1. Body Constitution

First the basic or birth constitution of the person must be determined. This is the main background factor in all treatment. The constitution is of seven types as already discussed: Vata, Pitta, Kapha, Vata-Pitta, Vata-Kapha, Pitta-Kapha and balanced Vata-Pitta-Kapha.

2. Disease Condition

Determination of the particular disease is the major object of the clinical examination. Under this heading, one has to assess the causative factors, aggravated doshas, affected bodily tissues, habitat, time, strength, signs and symptoms. As the strength of the disease can be assessed only by the consideration of this factor, the entire clinical examination is designed to elucidate its nature.

3. Tissue Vitality

The seven types of tissues - plasma, blood, muscle, fat, bone, marrow, and reproductive - are examined for the assessment of their optimal state along with the examination of the mind. A person having particular tissue vitality does not suffer from diseases affecting that tissue. Note the section on *Tissue Sara*.

4. Body Build

This refers to the compactness and tone of the tissues like bone, muscle, and blood. Generally, it means a well-built body in which the bones are symmetrical and well distributed, and in which the joints are well bound with enough flesh and blood. Such persons are strong; those who appear contrary, with weak or flaccid muscles and joints, are weak.

5. Body Measurement

Proper proportion of the body and limbs indicates health. Improper proportion shows disease. This factor has already been discussed under Measurement of Body Proportion.

6. Adaptability

Substances which are homologous, or of like nature to the body, are known as "Satmya." Individuals for whom ghee, milk, sesame oil and all the six tastes are adaptable are strong, tolerant of difficulties, and long lived. Those who have adapted to only a few things, who are hypersensitive or intolerant of many things, are generally weak and short lived.

This factor of adaptation is very important in health and disease. We easily habituate ourselves in life, including to health matters of food, exercise and medicines. If we are habituated to bad food, wrong exercise and to a poor health regimen, then our health will not be good. For this same reason, treatment takes time, as habits must change. Similarly, we should strive to create good habits in children so that they don't become habituated to what is harmful for them.

7. Mental Nature

The mind is the controller of the body as long as it is in contact with the soul. According to its degree of strength, the mind is graded as either high, medium or low. Accordingly, individuals have three types of mental constitutions according to the three gunas of Sattva, Rajas and Tamas. Those who are predominant in Sattva possess high mental strength. Those predominant in Tamas possess low mental strength. Those predominant in Rajas fall in the middle. Mental constitution has been described in detail elsewhere in this text.

8. Capacity for Food

The capacity for food is to be judged from the ability to ingest and digest food and by regularity of the appetite. Good capacity for food indicates health, while poor capacity shows disease. That is why loss of appetite or dislike of food is a common symptom of many diseases starting with the common cold.

9. Capacity for Exercise

The capacity for exercise is judged by the capacity for work. From the capacity for work, three degrees of strength - low, moderate and high - can be determined. Those who have fatigue upon slight exertion are low in strength. Those who do not fatigue even after severe exertion are high in strength. The rest fall in the middle.

10. Age

Age is broadly divided into three phases: Childhood, middle age and old age. Kapha, Pitta and Vata energies are more predominant during childhood, middle age and old age respectively. Diseases occurring in these age groups should consider the dosha governing that stage of life. Particularly for elderly people, Vata should always be considered in treatment, regardless of their birth constitution.

EIGHTFOLD PATIENT EXAMINATION

Probably the most important form of patient examination practiced in Ayurveda is the eightfold examination (Ashtavidha Pariksha). These provide a good idea about the nature of the illness and the condition of the patient. The eight factors examined are:

1. Pulse	2. Tongue	3. Voice	4. Skin
5. Eyes	6. General appearance	7. Urine	8. Stool

1. Examination of the Pulse

The term "nadi" literally means a tube or channel through which something flows. Texts dealing with Yoga philosophy use this term for the nerves. In the context of the eightfold examination, nadi refers to the arteries. Pulse examination (Nadi Pariksha) is the examination of the arterial pulses at certain points on the body.

The early hours of the morning are the best time for pulse examination. It can be misleading or incorrect if done after the patient has taken food, exercise or a bath, after taking intoxicants, having sex, sleep or when afflicted with hunger, thirst, anger, grief or worry.

The radial pulse at the wrist is best suited for examination. The pulse on the right hand is selected for men and on the left hand for women. The physician should place the first three fingers (index, middle and ring) of his right hand on the pulse at the wrist of the patient. The fingers of the physician should be placed softly but firmly so that even slight movements of the pulse can be felt. The examination is better done three times with an interval of several seconds in between.

The main factors to be noted during pulse examination are pulse rate (Spandana Samkhya), pulse character (Gati) and pulse qualities (Gunas). The pulse rate is the number of beats per thirty seconds (pala) or double the amount per minute as follows:

Newborn child	112 per minute
3 - 7 years	90 per minute
30 - 50 years	75 per minute

The pulse character is described as resembling the movement of certain animals and birds. Vata pulse is said to be like a snake, Pitta like a frog, and Kapha like a swan. Pulse qualities like warm, cold, soft, hard, thin, thick, full, empty, collapsed, volume and spiral movement can be ascertained by careful palpation.

Abnormal or Disease Pulse

- In conditions of Vata aggravation, the pulse resembles the movement of a snake or leech and is irregular, unsteady and neither hot nor cold.
- In Pitta conditions, it is like the movements of a frog, crow, sparrow, crane or quail, and is warm, rapid, thin and soft.
- In Kapha conditions, it is like the movement of a swan, pigeon, dove, cock, peacock, or elephant and is steady, cold, thick, and full or hard.

2. Examination of the Tongue

The tongue provides important information on the health of a person, particularly for the diagnosis of digestive disorders. By examining the tongue, one can infer the state of Vata, Pitta and Kapha, the plasma, blood and the digestive fire.

When Vata is high, the tongue is dry, rough and cracked. When Pitta is aggravated, the tongue is reddish in color with sores or ulcers and a burning sensation. During Kapha imbalances, the tongue becomes coated, white and slimy. In anemia, it loses its normal color and becomes white and smooth. When Agni is impaired, the tongue becomes coated with a white layer (Ama) that cannot be removed by washing or scraping, and the breath is usually unpleasant.

3. Examination of the Voice

The voice of a person reveals much about their strength and weakness and the doshas involved. It is particularly important for diseases of the head, throat and lungs, which often impair the vocal organs.

4. The Skin - Examination by Touch

This method is related to palpation and mainly notes normal or abnormal conditions through the skin. The skin is the largest organ in the body. It is closely connected to and reflects the conditions of Rasa Dhatu or the plasma. As the Rasa is the dominant bodily tissue, the skin reflects what is occurring in the body as a whole.

The skin of a person with a Pitta disorder is hot and a little oily, possibly inflamed. The skin of one with a Kapha disorder is cold and damp, and generally pale. The skin of one suffering from a Vata disease is cold, dry or rough, with possible darkish discolorations.

5. Examination of the Eyes

Examination of the eyes of a patient provides much information about the condition of the doshas. Red or inflamed eyes, along with sensitivity to bright lights or sunlight, reveal Pitta conditions. Kapha conditions are revealed by mucus in the eyes or by watering of the eyes along with cloudy vision. Vata problems manifest by dryness and tremors of the eyes.

6. General Appearance

The general appearance of the patient reveals much about their condition, including the luster of the skin or the posture of the person. Here also comes examination of the different systems of the body, which are looked at according to their function and external appearance. For many Ayurvedic doctors, this method is more important than pulse diagnosis. Each system, along with its relevant functions and organs, is examined in various ways, with reference particularly to the predominant doshas and the qualities of damaged or healthy tissues.

7. Examination of the Urine

Examination of the urine is a special diagnostic tool in Ayurveda. The urine sample should be collected in a clean vessel, preferably in a sterilized glass jar, tumbler or test-tube, taken directly at the time of urination after avoiding the first few drops.

Sesame Oil Drop Urine Examination –
Taila Bindu Pariksha

A small quantity of urine is taken in a broad-mouthed glass vessel and kept undisturbed in a place free from wind, sun and other disturbing factors. A moderate-sized drop of sesame oil is then taken with a stick and allowed to fall on the surface of the urine from a height of two or three inches, gently and without disturbing the urine. The condition of the oil drop should be carefully observed for its spread and the different shapes or patterns that it assumes. The following interpretations can be drawn from its observations:

Mode of Spread, Pattern, Shape, Conditions

High Vata	Floats like a boat; resembles a snake; lengthwise
High Pitta	Bubbles appear; splits into small drops; assumes the shape of an umbrella or ring
High Kapha	Stays like a pearl; resembles a sieve

8. Examination of the Stool

The stool provides information about the condition of the doshas, the tissues and the food digested both in healthy and diseased states. Hence, Ayurveda advocates its examination as a diagnostic tool, especially in disorders of the digestive and excretory systems.

If the digestion and absorption of food is normal, the stool is well formed and floats on water. This indicates that there is no Ama in the body. On the contrary, if digestion is not correct, the stool does not float on water but is slimy, with various colors, contains undigested food particles, and has a bad odor. This indicates Ama in the system. Examination of the stool can be carried out to check for abnormal blood or fat or for the presence of parasites.

EXAMINATION OF DISEASE – ROGA PARIKSHA

For proper diagnosis, the disease itself must be examined. We must determine the qualities, symptoms and sites of the disease. There are five approaches for this:

• Causative factors (Nidana)

- Preliminary symptoms (Purvarupa)
- Primary signs and symptoms (Rupa)
- Means of alleviation (Upashaya)
- Disease pathogenesis (Samprapti)

Pathogenesis has already been discussed. Upashaya requires some clarification. In certain diseases, diagnosis becomes difficult or may not even be possible. In such cases, the patient is given certain exploratory treatments in order to see how the disease responds to them. Such methods are called Upashaya or "means of alleviation". By trying out certain herbs or therapies on a patient and noting the response that occurs, we can get a better idea of their real condition and how to treat it in the long run.

The program of examination for the patient should consist of:

- Factors that aggravate the disease
- Causative factors
- Onset
- Location
- Pain
- Sound
- Touch
- Color
- Taste
- Signs and symptoms
- Complications
- Stage of aggravation
- Continuity of disease
- Lessening of disease
- Sequelae
- Name and classification of disease
- Medicines
- Rules of treatment
- Odor

The diagnosis of the particular disease is based upon these methods but Ayurveda also places a great emphasis on methods for determining the dosha behind the disease. These are useful for both the experienced and the beginning practitioner. In this respect, Charaka states:

"When classified according to cause, pain, color, site, form and nomenclature, the number of diseases becomes countless. A physician need not be ashamed if he is unable to name all diseases as there can be no definite standardization of nomenclature for disease."

The same provoked dosha produces various diseases according to its location, by which tissues it has entered into. For example, Vata entering into the blood causes gout, while entering into the bones causes arthritis. Therefore, treatment should be initiated after diagnosing the nature of the disease relative to the dosha and the tissue affected, as well as by other special factors. Merely to know the modern medical name for a disease is not enough to determine the appropriate Ayurvedic treatment.

The great complexity of diseases can be explained by imbalances of the three doshas. In this way, Ayurveda can treat diseases in a direct manner that goes right to the cause and does not become concerned with unnecessary details. Through understanding Vata, Pitta and Kapha along with their normal and abnormal states, we can understand and treat all possible diseases, even if we do not know their specific forms or manifestations. This is the great beauty and simplicity of Ayurveda, which makes it so enduring as a system of medicine. It places the key to health and disease in our own hands.

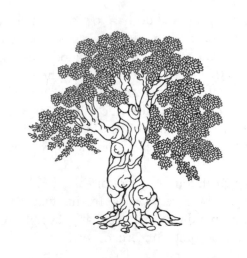

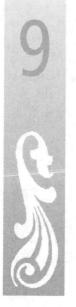

The Many Methods of Ayurvedic Treatment

He who knows only the theory but is not proficient in practice gets bewildered on confronting a patient, just as a coward feels afraid on the battlefield. Only the wise person who knows both theory and practice is capable of obtaining success, just as only a two-wheeled chariot is useful in the battlefield.

— *Sushruta*

Ayurvedic treatment is a comprehensive system for bringing into balance all the different aspects of our nature from the body to the soul. It is a complete life-science and life strategy that facilitates health so that we can employ all of our potentials in life. The main Ayurvedic term for treatment is Chikitsa, which derives from the root "kit", meaning the cure or relief from disease, the removal of its cause. The Ayurvedic definition of treatment is the widest possible for any system of medicine and includes all methods of healing from the physical to the spiritual. Ayurvedic treatment consists of the beneficial usage of herbs, diet and practices prescribed separately or together to eliminate both manifest and unmanifest diseases. These methods are described as:

• Contrary to the cause of the disease
• Contrary to the disease itself
• Contrary to both the cause and the disease
• Similar to the cause of disease
• Similar to the disease itself
• Similar to both the cause and the disease

Contrary treatment means prescribing food, herbs and lifestyle of opposite qualities to those of the disease, like taking hot potency herbs to counter diseases arising from cold. Similar treatment means prescribing herbs in small dosages that have qualities similar to the disease, which works on a subtle level, like giving a small amount of a toxic herb to counter the effects of a similar toxin or nervous disorder in the body.

These definitions cover the principles of allopathy, homeopathy, and naturopathy. That is why Ayurveda does not oppose any of these "pathies" and why it is called "the mother of all medical sciences".

Homeopathy, which means treatment by similars, and allopathy, meaning treatment by contraries, can be regarded, in the words of the founder of Homeopathy, Samuel Hahnemann, as "the exact opposite" of each other. But according to Ayurveda, both are acceptable alternative approaches. Thus, the homeopathic opium that cures constipation and the allopathic opium that causes it both fall within the range of Ayurvedic therapeutic measures.

The Ayurvedic definition of medicine is broad and comprehensive. "Nothing exists in the realm of thought or experience that cannot be used as a medicine (therapeutic agent)." This means that all existing phenomena, physical or psychological - including anger and tranquility; joy and sorrow; fear and confidence; love and hate; food and drink; medicinal substances of mineral, vegetable or animal origin; practices like fasting, massage, postures and exercises; desirable or undesirable experiences or situations; social, climatic or geographical conditions; laudatory or adverse comments; and good, bad or indifferent thoughts - have an important bearing on health. There is nothing that can be experienced or conceived of that does not influence the body or mind positively or negatively. Merely hearing the name of a friend or foe can affect the metabolism for better or for worse. Since anything that affects the constitution can be utilized as a therapeutic agent, everything is a medicine in one way or the other.

Ayurvedic treatment covers a vast field. It not only aims at relief from disease but also at bringing the patient back to his or her normal individual constitutional state. It includes relief from stress and strain, worry and anxiety. It consists not only of medicines, but also of guidelines for optimal diet, daily routine, environment and mental health.

The term Kaya-chikitsa refers specifically to Ayurvedic treatment. There are three main words for the body in Ayurveda: *Deha, sharira,* and *kaya.* Each has a specific meaning. Deha derives from the root "dih", which means "that which is nourished". Thus deha carries the sense of anabolism or growth. The term sharira is derived from the root "shri", meaning "that which decays". The word sharira carries the sense of catabolism or decline. The term kaya is derived from the root "chi" meaning "selection of suitable nutrition", the ability to absorb useful substances and eliminate non-useful ones. This carries the sense of both anabolism and catabolism, or metabolism. The process of metabolism takes place with the help of digestive juices, enzymes and hormones and so kaya also refers to Agni or the digestive fire. Thus, Kaya-chikitsa means the treatment of the whole body and of Agni, of digestion and metabolism.

Preventive Measures

Ayurveda emphasizes preventive measures, particularly as part of everyday living practices. The preventive aspects of Ayurveda consist of three main disciplines, which have already been discussed in detail.

The first is Personal Hygiene (Swastha Vritta), consisting of the appropriate daily routine, seasonal regimen, and ethical conduct. Swastha means a physically, psychologically and spiritually harmonious condition. Various methods that increase physical, mental, and spiritual strength come under this branch.

The second is Rasayana and Vajikarana, the use of the rejuvenative and invigorating agents. These are special herbs to prevent aging, strengthen immunity, improve mental faculties, and increase vitality. Vajikaranas are specifically used as aphrodisiacs and fertility-improving agents. Such practices require preliminary purification or Pancha Karma treatment for their full benefit to accrue.

The third is the practice of Yoga. Though Yoga in itself is a separate discipline from Ayurveda aimed at Self-realization, as a form of medicine, it is mainly considered as part of the rejuvenation (Rasayana) practice of Ayurveda. The regular practice of Yoga keeps both body and mind fit, which provides a sense of well-being, prevents aging, and inhibits disease from developing.

Dietetics – Pathyapathya

Diet is not only good for general health maintenance but also treats many diseases, in which case it is modified relative to each particular condition. Pathya means a diet and other regimens that create health and counter disease; Apathya means the contrary, that which is not appropriate and which aggravates disease. Ayurveda places a great emphasis on this principle. It says, "If a person uses Pathya (wholesome diet and life-regimes) there may be no need for medicine. If the patient indulges in Apathya, or the contrary, medicines, even if appropriate, will not work." A variety of dietetic preparations, largely of a vegetarian nature, are described in Ayurveda relative to different diseases. Note the section on food and diet in this regard.

Lifestyle – Vihara

Vihara refers to the daily practices and routines observed during health and disease. For example, during a fever, one should avoid sleep during the day, baths, oil massage, food, sexual activity, anger and excitement, exposure to wind, and exercise because such practices aggravate fevers. One should, on the contrary, take complete rest, keep the mind calm and at ease, fast, and so on. In this way, Vihara consists of lifestyle and psychological factors for treating disease. Ayurvedic doctors usually prescribe a particular lifestyle regimen not only relative to the constitution of the person but also relative to the particular diseases they might have. Most of these practices are simple and part of everyday living but others may involve special exercises, like particular Yoga postures, which require detailed instruction.

Psychosomatic Medicine

Ayurveda is a system of medicine with an inherent psycho-somatic orientation. The diagnosis and management of each patient is attended by a psychosomatic approach. No treatment is advised without keeping in view the mental nature of the patient, which forms a principal aspect of clinical considerations. The management of disease is advised in view of psychosomatic factors and their treatment through lifestyle, ethical regimen, meditation, mantra, and herbs to increase intelligence. The Ayurvedic doctor carefully monitors the psychological as well as the physical condition of the patient during the course of treatment, making sure the emotional side of the disease is properly considered along with the physical.

THREE LEVELS OF AYURVEDIC THERAPIES

Ayurveda recognizes three levels of therapies – rational, psychological and spiritual. Rational therapy is mainly for the treatment of physical diseases by physical treatment methods. Psychological therapy is for calming the mind and emotions and includes meditation. Spiritual therapy consists of yogic and occult methods to counter the effects of karma that prevent ordinary physical and psychological treatments from working.

- Rational or objectively planned therapy – Yukti Vyapashraya
- Psychological therapy – Sattvavajaya
- Spiritual therapy – Daiva Vyapashraya

Western medicine recognizes only a kind of rational therapy, the treatment of bodily conditions by objectively verifiable medicines. Ayurveda considers such an approach to be useful but incomplete, only one part of medicine. Without considering the role of the mind and of karma, we can neither understand nor properly treat the majority of diseases, which have subjective causes and complications.

Some scholars view Ayurveda as a rational system of medicine that arose historically out of primitive religio-magical roots, like the use of mantras and amulets giving way to herbs and surgery. However, Ayurveda has never separated itself off from these subtle and spiritual levels of healing. It also considers them to be rational but from the standpoint of our immortal soul, not merely that of the physical body. These remain an integral part of Ayurvedic treatment to the present day, which uses gems, mantras and rituals, as well as diet and herbs.

1. Rational Therapy

Rational or objectively planned therapy refers to the usage of specific medicines along with dietary regimens to counter the negative qualities evidenced by the disease. It is based upon logic and experience and reflects the Ayurvedic model for understanding the workings of natural forces in the body. Most Ayurvedic medical practice today falls within this field and it is specific to problems with a clearly defined physical origin and pathology. It generally consists of prescribing diet, herbs, exercise and lifestyle recommendations contrary to the doshic nature of the disease.

2. Psychological Therapy

Ayurvedic psychological therapy means controlling the mind to counter negative emotional states. It consists of developing the clear or Sattvic quality of the mind for gaining self-knowledge and freedom from desire. It uses the practices of Yoga and meditation to promote longevity, aid in rejuvenation, and treat disease, particularly mental disorders. It has a spiritual implication but relies less on ritualistic practices, as does spiritual therapy.

3. Spiritual Therapy

Spiritual, literally "celestial" therapy, is applied to diseases that are neither purely physical nor psychological and whose formation cannot be explained from evident causes. It consists of various subtle, religious or occult methods to ward off negative influences and to promote those which are positive. Such methods include chanting mantras, the spiritual use of herbs and gems, rituals for giving good fortune (Mangala), offerings of oblations (Bali), offerings in general (Upahara), fasting (Upavasa), pilgrimages (Gamana), performance of prostrations (Pranipata), fire sacrifices (Homa), ceremonial penances (Prayaschitta), and rituals for well-being (Swastyayana).

This therapy is found not only in Ayurveda but also in the tradition of Vedic Astrology (Jyotish) as well as in various yogic approaches, particularly teachings of the Tantric order. Much of it is considered to be magical in nature but it has its logic for countering negative karmic patterns. With these three different types of therapies, Ayurveda provides diverse methods and approaches for dealing with all possible difficulties in health and well-being.

The curative aspect of Ayurveda treats diseases and contains an entire range of therapeutic measures. These curative aspects also consist of three parts – Internal Medicine, External Medicine and Surgery – which are discussed in detail below. Most attention will be given to the Internal Medicine portion as it is the most important.

Internal Medicine

This is the main discipline of Ayurvedic medicine, the application of medicines for dealing with the diseases of the body. It consists of two primary procedures – Purification (Shodhana) and Palliation (Shamana).

Purification – Shodhana

Shodhana means radical purification that eliminates excess doshas from the body. As excess doshas are the primary cause of disease, this method is the most direct for curative purposes. It consists of the Five Purification practices of Pancha Karma therapy. These methods are explained separately under Pancha Karma and are the most significant of Ayurvedic clinical methods.

Palliation – Shamana

It is not always possible to treat diseases with Purification therapy because of various factors. Purification therapy can be very strong and is not suitable for weak or debilitated individuals. In such cases, a milder method is employed called Palliation. This means a gradual reduction of the aggravated doshas at their respective sites as a means of either curing the disease or decreasing its symptoms. Disease-causing doshas, when eliminated by Purification therapy (Shodhana), do not recur but chances of recurrence do exist under Palliation therapy. Palliation consists of seven parts:

Seven Methods of Palliation – Shamana

1. Kshut, literally "hunger" – fasting or light diet
2. Trit, literally "thirst" – restriction of fluid intake
3. Vyayama – exercise of various types
4. Atapa-sevana – sunbathing
5. Maruta-sevana – fresh air and exposure to the wind
6. Dipana – herbs that increase digestive power
7. Ama-pachana – herbs that destroy Ama or toxins

These methods reduce the accumulated doshas, eliminate toxins and cleanse the channels for a smooth flow of energy. They are a helpful preliminary practice to Purification therapy and are a useful part of health maintenance for cleansing the digestive system.

PALLIATION FOR VATA

Vata people often do not possess the physical stamina for stronger purification therapies and so are more likely to require Palliation methods. Vata aggravation arises either owing to deficient nutrition (Dhatukshaya) or obstruction in the channels (Margavarodha), as already noted. Vata also gets disturbed when Ama is mixed with it and is then called Sama Vata. Palliation therapy is indicated for Sama Vata or for Vata aggravation owing to malnutrition, both of which are caused by weakness in the digestive system. However, it employs different methods in each case.

For Sama Vata, the therapy focuses on herbs to burn up Ama (Ama-pachana) like dry ginger and black pepper, along with herbs to increase the digestive fire (Agni-dipana) like fennel or calamus. Mild exercise is indicated with calming Yoga postures, like sitting poses. Short- term fasting or a light diet may be recommended as well.

For Vata aggravated by malnutrition, Palliation consists of tonification (Brimhana) or building therapy. Here an adequate nutritious diet is indicated, consisting of wheat, rice, sweet fruit, root vegetables, dairy products, raw sugar, oils like sesame, and nuts like almonds along with tonic herbs like ashwagandha or bala. For this type of high Vata, it is said, "Tonification is as good as Palliation" (see section on *Tonification* in this regard).

PALLIATION FOR PITTA

Pitta accumulates owing to the increase of hot and sharp qualities in the body. At such times, the patient should be massaged with cooling oils like sandalwood prepared in a coconut oil base. Light exercise is good, like swimming in cool water, and a cool and light diet is indicated with ghee, sweet fruit, wheat and mung beans, along with relaxation. Bitter herbs like gentian and aloe, along with mild spices like cloves, coriander or turmeric, help burn up toxins and increase digestive capacity.

In some conditions, like long-lasting fevers, Pitta causes an increase of dryness in the body. Here one must remember that this dryness is not the original quality of Pitta but a side effect of the high heat that overcomes the lesser damp quality of Pitta. For such conditions the best Palliation therapy is to give ghee prepared with bitter herbs like katuka or barberry.

PALLIATION FOR KAPHA

Kapha types suffer from low digestive power and slow metabolism. For Palliation, Kapha requires strong digestive stimulants like trikatu, chitrak, cayenne, turmeric and dry ginger. Fasting for longer periods of time without food or water is good, followed by a light and dry diet. Strong physical exercise, reduction of sleep, exposure to sun, wind and heat, and stronger yogic practices including Yoga Kriyas can be carried out as well, but with adequate care not to overly weaken the patient. Palliation for Kapha usually consists of stronger practices owing to the inherent strength of Kapha constitution.

THE SIX MAIN METHODS OF TREATMENT – SHAD-UPAKRAMAS

Three opposite pairs of Ayurvedic treatment approaches exist, six in total, marking the entire field of therapeutics:

1. Reduction – Langhana
2. Tonification – Brimhana

3. Drying – Rukshana
4. Oleation – Snehana

5. Sudation – Swedana
6. Astringent – Stambhana

The first method of each pair, Reduction, Drying and Sudation (sweating) methods, reduces excess factors in the body - Kapha and excess body tissues. The second of each pair, Tonification, Oleation and Astringent methods, increases deficient body tissues such as are commonly created by Vata disorders.

For diseases owing to lack of proper nutrition like low body weight, low energy and improper growth of the body, Tonification, Oleation, and Astringent methods are appropriate. For diseases arising from excessive nutrition of the body like obesity, atherosclerosis, hypertension and Ama conditions, Reduction, Drying and Sudation forms of treatment are required.

1. REDUCTION – Langhana

Many of us suffer from overweight or toxicity that must be reduced or eliminated for health and vitality to be restored. Such excess conditions underlie many diseases, particularly those involving congestion or fever. The therapy that produces lightness of the body by reducing such disease-causing excesses is called Langhana. This type of therapy is indicated for high Kapha and Pitta, for diseases caused by Ama and weak digestion, for excess of poor quality tissues like fat, muscle and bone, and for toxins in the blood. Whenever there is an excess of waste products in the body, Reduction therapy is also advised. Charaka explains a similar type of therapy under the heading "Asantarpana", described as following strict dietary restrictions of Reduction therapy for long periods of time, along with hard work, vigorous exercise, and giving up of comforts.

Reduction therapy consists of two parts – Palliation (Shamana) and Purification (Shodhana) – already described as the two main procedures of Ayurvedic internal medicine.

Langhana consists of ten methods. The first four are four types of Purification processes. The remaining six are Palliation methods.

Methods of Reduction

1. Vamana (emetics)	2. Virechana (purgation)
3. Asthapana Basti (decoction enemas)	4. Shiro-virechana (cleansing nasal medications)
5. Restriction of fluid intake (Trit)	6. Exposure to wind or fresh air (Maruta-sevana)
7. Sunbathing (Atapa-sevana)	8. Taking of herbs to promote digestion (Ama-pachana)
9. Fasting	10. Exercise including Yoga postures

2. TONIFICATION – Brimhana

Many people suffer from low energy, low body weight, weak immune function and fatigue that requires restoring strength and rebuilding bodily tissues. Tonification therapy is the reverse of Reduction. The line of treatment, which increases body weight and strength, is called Brimhana, or bulk increasing. This therapy is indicated for the emaciated, weak or debilitated, and for those in convalescence from chronic illnesses like anemia, malabsorption, tuberculosis, or other wasting diseases. It is essential for Vata disorders that originate from malnutrition. It is useful in many Pitta and some Kapha conditions that also weaken the tissues. It is contraindicated in conditions of Ama or toxins, and during febrile diseases.

Tonification therapy consists of a rich diet, tonic herbs, rest and a relaxing lifestyle. Food prepared with ghee, butter, sesame oil, milk, raw sugar and jaggery is used. Almonds, pistachios, cashews and other nuts should be added. Tonic herbs like shatavari, ashwagandha, bala, ginseng, and amalaki are specific, particularly the herbal jellies (Prash and Avaleha) prepared from them. The lifestyle should have no tension or stress, with plenty of rest and enjoyment. For Tonification, the herbs indicated under rejuvenation (Rasayana) and invigoration (Vajikaranas) are also good. Mental tranquility should be maintained throughout the course of treatment.

Tonification According To Dosha

VATA individuals require strong tonification. For this, warm sesame oil massage, warm baths, warm clothing, and a warm environment and climate are essential. Nutritive food is indicated with dairy products, grains like wheat and oats, nuts, and raw sugars. Tonic herbs like ashwagandha and bala should be taken along with herbs to increase the digestive fire like trikatu or ginger to help digest them.

PITTA people require moderate tonification. They should receive massage with cooling oils like coconut. The diet should consist of cooling and nourishing food like mung beans, wheat, basmati rice, raw vegetables and sweet dairy products, including ghee. Fasting and the use of hot spices are not good in their case. In severe cases, all spices must be avoided.

KAPHA people require the minimum tonification. As their appetite is not strong, they should eat whole grains like basmati rice, barley, or corn, with a lot of spices like trikatu, cayenne, or garlic, and drink herbal wines (Asavas and Arishtas) made from ashwagandha or bala, or take tonic herbs like garlic or shilajit.

3. DRYING METHOD – Rukshana

Rukshana means the therapy by which the oily, sticky and fatty constituents of the body are dried up and reduced. It eliminates excess mucus, fat and water from the tissues and organs. For this purpose, food with drying qualities are used. This includes grains like barley and rye, beans like soy and horse gram, and honey that is over six months old. Dry massage with powders of calamus, sandalwood, lodhra, or udumbara is used to remove oiliness from the skin. Decoctions of Dashamula or astringent herbs like catechu are taken internally.

Drying method is indicated for diseases in which Kapha increases due to liquification, as in the common cold, cough with expectoration and diabetes. It counters excess fluids and secretions and reduces congestion.

4. OLEATION – Snehana

Oleation therapy is the reverse of Drying therapy. Snehana renders dry or depleted bodily constituents oily or unctuous. Oleation is carried out with four main general types of oils: Ghee (clarified butter), vegetable oils (like sesame), muscle fat and bone marrow. Oleation can be administered orally through food and drink, through the rectum by the use of enemas and through the skin by massage.

This therapy is indicated for Vata diseases owing to dryness, and as in some cases as under Palliation, for Pitta aggravation due to heat and dryness. Oleation therapy is divided into two types: External and internal.

External Oleation

External oleation consists of different types of oil massage appropriate for different constitutions as already outlined under Palliation therapy. Usually Kapha-type people require the least amount of oleation. In their case, massage is better with heating herbs like calamus or camphor that are mixed in a rubbing alcohol base. External oil massage is known in Ayurveda as "Abhyanga", and has already been described under Daily Regimens.

Internal Oleation

This is divided into three types:

• Palliating (Shamana), which is included Palliation therapy;
• Purifying (Shodhana), oleation performed preliminarily to Pancha Karma or Purification therapy;
• Brimhana or tonifying.

For high Vata conditions, tonifying Oleation therapy is excellent and is one of the best ways of immediately lowering Vata. For Pitta and Kapha, medicated oils should be used internally for Palliation. In this regard, sesame oil is best for Vata, ghee for Pitta, and mustard oil for Kapha. Tonifying oleation therapy requires applying large amounts of oil internally and externally with due regard not to weaken the digestive fire or to suppress the appetite of the person.

5. SUDATION – Swedana

Sweating is well known for its cleansing value for the skin and the blood and for countering cold. Swedana means the procedure to induce sweating or perspiration. It may be brought about by heat or fire (with Agni) or without application of heat (Niragni Sweda). There are four types of Swedana where heat is necessary:

• Tapa Sweda – application of dry heat, like heating pads or hot sand;

- Ushma Sweda – application of steam;
- Apanaha Sweda – application of hot poultices like wheat flour;
- Drava Sweda – use of hot liquids or herbal decoctions externally for baths.

These four are further divided into fourteen types according to the methods and articles used. Heat may be created indirectly through exercise, blankets, sun bathing, or the drinking of herbal wines.

Sudation therapy is indicated for diseases that result from cold and dampness, and those in which poorly formed bodily tissues are in excess. It is divided into external and internal types.

External Sweating Therapy

This therapy is further divided into either whole-body or partial-body therapies (Sarvanga and Ekanga Sweda). It is used mainly for high Vata and Kapha, which are aggravated by cold or damp qualities. For high Pitta, this therapy should generally be avoided.

For whole-body sweating therapy for Vata, one should use the medicated steam of anti-Vata herbs like Dashamula, rasna, and nirgundi. For this a special apparatus, or sweat box, is prepared in which the patient can lie or sit comfortably with his head on the outside so it does not get too hot. For Kapha patients, anti-Kapha herbs are used for the steam like lodhra, calamus, or eucalyptus, which are hot and dry in nature. Generally, before carrying out an external sweating therapy, a light oil massage should be given. For Kapha, massage with hot, dry herbs like calamus or mustard, again preferably in a rubbing alcohol base, is best.

Partial-body sweating can be done in various ways. For Kapha diseases, dry fomentation with sand can be used, or exposure to infrared lamps. For Vata, Nadi Swedana is used. In this the medicated steam of anti-Vata herbs like Dashamula is directed through a hose (nadi), which is used to foment a particular part of the body. This is done by hooking up a plastic hose to the top of a pressure cooker in which the herbs are cooking and directing the steam through it.

Internal Sweating Therapy

This is not always as effective as the external method but is easier to do. For this purpose, herbs with a hot nature and diaphoretic action are taken, like trikatu, ginger, cinnamon, or bayberry. Much of the Western and Chinese usage of diaphoretic herbs comes under this type of therapy, like taking hot ginger tea to promote sweating in order to relieve the common cold.

6. ASTRINGENT METHOD – Stambhana

Astringent means contracting, tightening or preventing unwanted discharges. The procedure by which the flow of fluids in the body is lessened or checked is called Stambhana, which literally means "stopping." This therapy is indicated in conditions where body fluids like water, blood, urine, feces, sweat, and plasma leave the body in abnormal amounts, resulting in debility. Such excess discharges manifest as excess sweating, running of the nose, bleeding, or diarrhea.

For diarrhea, intestinal astringents (Grahi) are used. First hot and pungent herbs are employed until the Ama or toxic food mass is digested. For example, first an Ama-burning herb like dry ginger is used and only then a more typical astringent like kutaj or alum root. For excess urination (polyuria) as in the case of diabetes, urinary astringents like lodhra are used. For excess bleeding or hemorrhage, hemostatic and styptic herbs are used, like turmeric or saffron. In tuberculosis and other wasting diseases of the lungs, plasma (Rasa Dhatu) leaves the body through the phlegm. In such conditions, Sitopaladi churna with a large amount of Vamsharochana (Bamboo manna) is good.

The Astringent method also counteracts the side effects of excess Sudation therapy, which can result in too much sweating. At such times, a cold shower or bath, sleeping in the cool air or moonlight, and taking coral or pearl powder internally is useful to stop sweating.

External Medicine – Bahya Parimarjana

External medicine consists of various procedures done externally to the patient. Besides internal medicine, there are extensive external therapies in Ayurveda in the form of oleation, sudation, baths, massage, different kinds of medicated gargles, application of pastes, application of powders, and other kinds of therapeutic procedures for the treatment of different kinds of ailments. Such treatments are as popular and effective today as in ancient times. We have described them under their appropriate places while considering the practices of internal medicine.

Surgery – Shastra Pranidhana

Classical Ayurveda contains a well-planned and systematic surgical discipline that considers all aspects of surgical practice. Ayurvedic texts, particularly *Sushruta Samhita*, describe a large variety of sharp and blunt instruments, splints and bandages for local applications. This has been discussed briefly under the Eight Branches of Ayurveda.

Assessment of Treatment

Treatment must bring about certain improved results in the patient to be regarded as successful. The above-mentioned methods of treatment are employed relative to several principles of which the following are most important: Constitution (Prakriti), age, adaptability (satmya), status of the doshas, tissues, waste-materials, Agni, channel systems, and Ojas of the patient. The specific medicines, their dosages and modes of administration are suitably selected in each individual case depending upon such relevant factors. The degree of success of treatment can be measured by the following indications:

Relief from the pain of the disease

Improvement of voice and complexion

Normalization of body weight

Increase in strength and vitality

Desire for food and improved appetite

Relish or taste for food while eating

Timely and proper digestion

Sleep at the proper time

Absence of fearful dreams or disturbed sleep

Feeling of happiness and vitality upon awakening

Proper elimination of urine, stool, and flatus

Lack of impairment of mind and senses

10 *Ayurvedic Clinical Procedures: Pancha Karma*

THE NEED FOR DETOXIFICATION

Many different detoxification programs are available today through different natural healing systems. One can undergo a round of colonics, take a liver flush, go to a sweat lodge or a steam bath, fast, take green juices or blood-purifying herbs, or any number of methods. Herbal approaches exist which systematically aim at cleansing all the main organs of the body. Most of us have been engaged in such therapies and have experienced various degrees of benefit from them, sometimes greatly so. Some of us have been weakened by them, occasionally to a significant degree.

Toxin has become a catchword for every sort of harmful substance that can accumulate in the body. Various and mysterious toxins have been blamed for all our health problems, and often with good reason. Whatever health problem we have will likely be accompanied by some sort of toxin, whether it be a bacteria, virus, yeast, a pollutant like heavy metals or pesticides, residue of drugs we have taken or, above all, the toxic remnants of bad diet and poor digestion. Such toxins not only cause disease but also are produced by disease and keep the disease process in motion.

There is no wonder that we feel toxic given the lack of quality today in our food, water, and air. Most of our food is old, over-processed and devitalized, containing various inorganic additives and contaminants. Our water is chemically treated and stale, unpleasant to the taste. Our air contains various chemicals and industrial wastes. If the quality of life is measured by the quality of these three main supports of life – our food, water and air – our life today is declining in all that really matters. Our artificial civilization has damaged the very biosphere in which we live and move. This must adversely affect our individual health and human life as well as the state of the planet.

Our dietary habits themselves are poor, so that whatever we eat may become hard to digest. Few people today cook or even know how to cook. Our meals are irregular, hurried and eaten with little attention. For the lack of real taste and vitality in our food, we substitute sugars, salt and spices, which jade our senses and derange our appetite yet further. We also lack in proper exercise or proper sleep and do not know how to conserve our energy, which we waste through various forms of indulgence and distraction.

We pollute our minds with artificial sensations through the low quality entertainment that we open ourselves up to via television, movies and pop music. On top of this may be a mental and emotional toxicity brought about through wrong relationships, stressful jobs and lifestyles, or lack of spiritual orientation in life. These psychological strains also trigger physical malfunctioning.

We are all suffering from toxins. They may not actually result in diagnosable diseases but they do impair our functioning, dull our minds and reduce our longevity. Such toxins are behind the rapid increase in chronic and difficult to treat conditions like allergies, immune system disorders, arthritis, chronic fevers, and chronic fatigue. They contribute to nervous and psychological conditions like insomnia, irritability, depression and anxiety. They are among the main causative factors for the primary modern fatal diseases of heart attacks and cancer.

Such toxins in the body are indicated by poor absorption, indigestion, gas and bloating, constipation, congestion, swollen glands, skin rashes, frequent colds and flus, and weak immune function. If we have a discernable tongue coating, bad breath, mucus in our system, tiredness when we get up in the morning, and lack of stamina physically, while psychologically we lack patience, peace and concentration, it is likely that we have such toxins in our system, perhaps at a deep level.

Allopathic medicine aims at the elimination of pathogens, which are also toxins of a kind, defined as various bacteria or viruses. It regards these external pathogens as the cause of disease rather than the wrong food, water, air, lack of exercise or improper lifestyle and the internal toxins created by such things, which allow us to be effected by these external forces. Bacteria and viruses require some sort of toxic accumulation in the body in which to grow. However, allopathic medicine does not have cleansing methods to remove these accumulations. It employs antibiotics to kill the bacteria and viruses that breed in them. The un-eliminated toxic mass then must breed more such pathogens. Such a method is like trying to sterilize a garbage heap rather than clean it up and remove it.

It is clear therefore that natural detoxification measures are necessary and essential for health in our environment today. It is also clear that among the smorgasbord of the available detoxification therapies there is much that is ill defined, one-sided, and which has potential side effects. How do we know which of these therapies we need? What are we detoxifying in ourselves and why? As all detoxification therapies are reducing, and to some extent therefore debilitating, if we are already weak, do we have the energy to support such procedures? And what do we do once we have detoxified ourselves? Is that the end? Do we go back to a life out of balance or is there a new way that we can orient our existence?

AYURVEDIC DETOXIFICATION

Ayurveda contains perhaps the most complex and specific

science of detoxification in natural medicine, an entire set of cleansing therapies called Pancha Karma, the five purificatory measures. These include oil massage, sweating therapies, enemas, purgatives, and the use of emetics given in a specific order, along with certain dietary regimens per individual constitution and disease conditions.

According to Ayurveda, we are all naturally healthy. Health is the natural state in which we keep our energies balanced through right interaction with our environment. Disease arises from outside contaminants that we get by opening ourselves up to harmful substances from the external world, through both the material substances that we take in through the body, and the impressions that we take in through the mind. Once these external factors are eliminated, our natural health and equilibrium will reassert itself of its own accord, unless it has already been severely damaged.

Generally, all toxins begin with Ama, defined in Ayurveda as the residue of poorly digested food that arises from eating heavy food like meat and dairy products, and oily, sweet, salty and sour food in general, such as abounds in the standard American diet. Ama has a sticky and heavy nature and lodges itself in the tissues where it ferments and causes poor tissue formation. Environmental toxins also weaken the digestive process and contribute to the formation of Ama, getting mixed along with it as undigestible substances.

Pancha Karma, which means a five-fold Purification therapy, is a special form of radical cleansing treatment in Ayurveda. It is perhaps the most important clinical procedure in Ayurveda because it is the best method to permanently eliminate excess doshas from the body. Pancha Karma is a great practice to eliminate the root of disease. Its five methods are:

THE FIVE METHODS OF PANCHA KARMA

1. Vamana	Herb induced emesis
2. Virechana	Herb induced purgation
3. Asthapana Basti	Medicated decoction enema

| 4. Anuvasana Basti | Medicated oil enema |
| 5. Nasya | Nasal intake of medication |

According to Sushruta, Rakta-moksha or therapeutic blood-letting is included instead of Asthapana Basti.

Action of Pancha Karma

Day and night during the digestive process, the doshas move into the gastrointestinal tract (Koshtha) from the tissues (Shakha). The body naturally tries to discard unwanted substances with these gastrointestinal secretions. Certain portions of the digestive tract are the main sites of secretion for the doshas: The stomach for Kapha, the small intestine for Pitta, and the large intestine for Vata. Pancha Karma enhances this natural process of the appearance of the doshas in certain parts of the gastrointestinal tract. Excess doshas are removed from the body through their respective digestive secretions.

As the doshas and tissues (Dhatus) are related to each other, these elimination procedures affect the tissues indirectly by removing the doshas that damage them.

- Elimination of Kapha by herb induced emesis causes an effect on the nutrient tissue-fluid pool, containing water and electrolytes, plasma, muscles and fat.
- Elimination of Pitta by purgation causes an indirect effect on the total coloring material in the body, particularly the blood and bile.
- Basti, medicated enema, contains warm oleating substances meant to nullify excess Vata. During the oil's contact with the membrane of the large intestine, it separates the sticky layers of solid fecal matter and, by enhancing better absorption, ultimately nourishes all the tissues.
- Nasal medications (Nasya) clean the sinuses and improve the function of the brain and sense organs.

Pancha Karma promotes the body's natural methods of eliminating unwanted substances. Its techniques are designed to take advantage of these phases of greater secretion or absorption at related mucous membrane sites.

OBJECTIVE OF PANCHA KARMA

Pancha Karma is used to achieve the three objectives of health maintenance, to treat disease and to prepare for rejuvenation.

Health Maintenance

Pancha Karma is recommended for most individuals, even those who are healthy, as part of regular seasonal regimens. The doshas naturally accumulate owing to seasonal changes and can cause disease if they are not removed.

- In the autumn or Vata season, Basti or medicated enema is advised to alleviate the normal aggravation of Vata caused by the wind and dryness of the season.
- In the spring or Kapha season, Vamana or Emesis is prescribed to remove excess Kapha caused by the coolness and dampness of the season.
- In summer or Pitta season, purgation is given to remove excess Pitta, caused by the season's heat.

Treatment of Disease

Pancha Karma is one of the main Ayurvedic methods of treating diseases, whether acute or chronic. This procedure should be carried out according to the excess doshas prevalent in the particular disease. In acute diseases, if the doshas are removed at the proper time, the disease attack can be immediately arrested. In chronic diseases, various toxins stick to the organs and cells. Unless these toxins and excess doshas are first removed by Pancha Karma therapies, other treatments cannot benefit the patient.

Preparation for Rejuvenation or Virilization Therapies

Pancha Karma is the main detoxification procedure that is done preliminarily to the application of rejuvenation and virilization therapies. Both these therapies are selective tissue-enriching programs. To achieve their best results, the body must be first purified. Once the excess doshas are removed, the bodily tissues can be revitalized in a direct manner. Otherwise, these revitalizing therapies can aggravate latent toxins and cause diseases.

PREPARATORY PRACTICES FOR PANCHA KARMA- PURVA KARMA

Pancha Karma is a clinical practice that requires a well-trained technician with extensive study and practice. Here we will outline the method and its main procedures so that the reader can understand its usefulness. Pancha Karma is a strategic detoxification therapy that must be prepared in the right manner. In order to remove excess doshas from the body, these must be first brought to the appropriate sites where they can be eliminated. These sites are the stomach for Kapha, the small intestine for Pitta, and the large intestine for Vata. To achieve this, two preparatory practices are recommended, Oleation and Sudation (Snehana and Swedana). Through these two procedures, the doshas localized in the tissues and skin are brought to the gastrointestinal tract where they can be eliminated.

Oleation therapy makes the main procedures of Pancha Karma less exhausting to the patient through the soothing effect of the oil on the tissues. The gastrointestinal tract, which has to produce more secretions in order to eliminate the doshas, benefits by the additional oil in the body. During Sudation or sweating therapy, the channels, openings and pores of the body are widened so that the doshas can move easily through them into the gastrointestinal tract for elimination. Sudation helps liquefy the doshas so that they drain into the digestive tract with minimal resistance. Oleation works to protect the tissues, loosening the doshas that are sticking to the walls of minute channels, creating a centripetal force. Sudation liquefies the doshas and opens the channels and pores for the movement of the doshas into the gastrointestinal tract.

Oleation – Snehana

A unique feature of Ayurveda is its use of oil therapies both to treat disease and as part of health maintenance. It is also applied as part of the preliminary practices of Pancha Karma. Oleation or oil therapy consists of the application of various oily substances either internally or externally. Ghee (clarified butter) and sesame oil are the two main oils used for this purpose. They are selected according to constitution, disease and predominance of the doshas. For Vata conditions, sesame oil is usually chosen and for Pitta and Kapha, ghee is used.

Light diet or fasting is recommended during oleation so that the food does not interfere with the oil in its lubricating action. Oleation is done on a daily schedule of gradually increasing dosage, using progressively more oil, until the signs of optimum oleation appear on the body. These are as follows:

- Oily appearance of skin (without any oil being externally applied)
- No white marks appearing after scratching the skin
- Disgust for oleating substances by the patient
- Appearance of oil in the stool, along with softness of the stool
- Appearance of lightness in the body

The initial oral dose for Oleation is 25 grams, about an ounce, the quantity that can be digested within six hours. This is the minimum dosage. The medium dosage is 37.5 grams, about an ounce and a half, the quantity that can be digested within twelve hours. Fifty grams, nearly two ounces, the quantity that can be digested within twenty-four hours, is regarded as the maximum dosage. According to the original dryness or oiliness of the digestive tract, the period required to achieve optimum oleation varies from three to seven days. In Ayurveda today, external oleation is done using liberal amounts of oil, usually sesame oil, on a special massage table by special Ayurvedic technicians. This is done daily for a period of about six days. Ghee may be taken internally during this period.

Sudation – Swedana

Sudation is a therapy by which a person is made to sweat. Sweating is a way of eliminating toxins from the body and is used to treat various diseases, like colds and flus, or as a health maintenance measure such as in saunas and sweat baths. Pancha Karma applies it in a special way as part of its greater strategy. Generally, it is done after Oleation and helps remove excess oil from the body. It has four types:

• By direct application of heat with electrical fomentation pads, or by heated cloth, sand, wheat flour, or salt in bandage form.

• By applying medicated poultices. This method is comparable to antiphlogistic treatment.

• By steam such as in a steam bath. The only difference is that the steam should be prepared from medicated herbs.

• By having the patient take a bath in which hot decoctions of various herbs are mixed with the water.

In Ayurveda today, generally a special steam box is employed and various Ayurvedic herbs that have sweat-inducing properties, like Dashamula or eucalyptus leaves, are used for the steam. After Sudation is completed, the patient should be given a light massage and bath and then should take a short rest. Not all the oil from the Oleation therapy will be removed through Sudation. For this reason, people undergoing Pancha Karma will often have oil in their hair, which will only wash out after a few days.

Primary Practices of Pancha Karma - Pradhana Karma

Once the preliminary procedures of Pancha Karma are completed, the primary practices are selected according to the nature of the person, disease and season. A patient may require several Pancha Karma procedures or one alone may be sufficient, depending upon their condition.

1. Emesis - Vamana

Emesis, or therapeutic vomiting, is the therapy of choice to eliminate excess Kapha from the body, removing it from the stomach through the mouth. It also helps relieve excess Pitta which sometimes moves upward into the stomach as well. The herb of choice for this procedure is Randia dumetorum seed, called emetic nut. Commonly, a mixture of this herb with calamus and licorice is used. In the West, licorice itself is easier to get. Salt water can also be used, which becomes emetic with high concentrations.

Indications and Contraindications

Vamana is indicated in Kapha predominant diseases like cough, asthma, repeated colds, dyspnea, diabetes, nausea, loss of appetite, indigestion and in certain nervous diseases like epilepsy caused by Kapha blocking the channels. It is contraindicated for young children, the elderly, the debilitated, very weak patients, and those with stomach ulcers, trauma to the lungs, heart disease and abdominal tumors as the patient must have sufficient strength to undergo the treatment.

Procedure

First the patient receives a course of Oleation and Sudation (Snehana and Swedana). Then, prior to the main treatment day, he should take Kapha-aggravating food like basmati rice with yogurt. Due to the preparatory treatment, the accumulated Kapha situated in the distant channels is loosened and moves back to the stomach. Then the patient sits on a low stool and his body is covered with a clean towel. He drinks 1 to 3 liters of a warm decoction of licorice tea. This secretion-promoting herb increases the bulk of the stomach contents.

Then the patient is given the main medicine to provoke vomiting. For this, calamus powder, licorice and the powder of the seeds of Randia dumetorum – each 1 gram – is taken with honey. This is a strong secretion-promoting mixture, which further stimulates Kapha to enter the gastrointestinal tract, as indicated by perspiration on the forehead. Vomiting starts shortly and the excess doshas, mainly Kapha but also some

Pitta, are eliminated from the body.

When the patient feels the sensation of nausea, he is instructed to vomit without undue strain. The head should be supported while the patient is actually vomiting. First the patient will vomit white, sticky and slimy substances (Kapha) and then yellow bile (Pitta) comes out. At this stage, vomiting usually stops automatically. The amount of vomit is evaluated as to whether it is maximum, medium, or minimum. These are judged from the number of vomitings and the total quantity of vomit expelled during the therapy.

Number of Vomitings, Quantity Expelled

Minimum - 325 cc.	Moderate - 650 cc.	Maximum - 1,300 cc.

However, the symptoms of proper elimination are more important than the quantity expelled or the number of vomitings. These are a feeling of lightness in the body, increased digestive power, decrease in the symptoms of the disease for which the emesis was prescribed, and the automatic stopping of vomiting after the expulsion of the doshas.

After treatment, the patient should clean up and take a short rest. Then he may smoke a mixture of medicated herbs and resins for removing residual Kapha in the upper respiratory tract. When he feels hungry, he should take a bath. Then starting with kicharee or basmati rice, he should slowly take a diet of increasingly heavier quality food, in such a way that on the seventh day he can return to his normal diet.

2. PURGATION – Virechana

The use of purgatives, or herbs to create strong evacuation of the bowels, is a well-known part of herbal treatment for many diseases including certain febrile conditions. In Ayurveda it is used mainly for the elimination of excess Pitta, though it can help remove Kapha as well. For this procedure, the patient is first given the usual Oleation and Sudation therapies (Snehana-Swedana). Purgation can be done three days after emesis, but it can be given directly if emesis is not required.

Indications and Contraindications

Purgation is indicated in skin diseases, chronic fevers, enlargement of the liver and spleen, jaundice, erysipelas, glandular swelling due to toxic blood, and various diseases of the blood due to high Pitta, like stomatitis, glossitis, and hyperacidity. It is contraindicated in the case of young children, very old and weak patients, when there has been bleeding through the rectum, ulcers in the large intestine, fissures in the anal canal, diarrhea or dysentery. The patient must have sufficient strength to undergo the treatment.

Procedure

The Ayurvedic medicine of choice in this therapy is a decoction of raisins, aragwadha and haritaki, 12 grams each, and katuka, 6 grams. First make a decoction of these herbs and then mix two ounces of this decoction with two ounces of castor oil. This is an ideal medicine for purgation. Among Western herbs, rhubarb root is particularly useful. It can be taken as a powder in dosages of 5 - 10 grams along with a quarter of that amount of cardamom or some other mild spice.

Purgation should be given four to six hours after sunrise. The patient drinks the purgative medicine first thing in the morning. Soon purgation starts due to the herbal secretion-promoting action. Three degrees of purgation have been described:

Purgation – Motions, Expelled Quantity

Minimum - 500 cc.	Moderate - 1,000 cc.	Maximum - 1,600 cc.

Indications of proper purgation are a feeling of cleanliness in the channels and sense organs, lightness in the body, and increase in appetite (after some time). During the procedure, the patient first passes liquid fecal matter and urine, then mucus (Kapha), and finally yellowish colored Pitta (bile). After treatment the patient should rest. Then, as in Vamana therapy, light food can be taken. This consists of starting with a light diet like vegetable soup and then slowly increasing the diet to a heavier quality, so that on the seventh day the patient can return to his normal diet. On the ninth day, Basti treatment can be started, if necessary.

3. - 4. MEDICATED ENEMAS – Basti

Enemas cleanse the large intestine. In Ayurveda, this therapy is employed in Pancha Karma to eliminate excess Vata once it has already been brought back to the large intestine by the appropriate preparatory measures. In this procedure, medicated oils and decoctions are introduced into the large intestine with the help of an enema bag. The word Basti means the urinary bladder. In ancient times, the urinary bladders of various dead animals were used for this purpose.

Four Ways of Classifying Enemas

1. According to the site where they are applied

Rectum	Vagina	Urethra	A wound cavity

2. According to the substance used

Cleansing (Niruha)	Oleating (Anuvasana)

In Niruha Basti, salt, honey, oils, pastes and decoctions of herbs are used. This is also known as Asthapana Basti. According to the variation of substances used, this Basti is further classified into Yapana, Brimhana, and so on. In Anuvasana Basti, only sesame oil or medicated sesame oil is used.

3. According to therapeutic action

Shodhana for Purification	Lekhana for reducing excess tissues
Snehana for Oleation	Brimhana for increasing deficient tissues in the body
Shamana for Palliation	Doshahara to remove particular doshas

4. According to the course of treatment

- Karma – Total course of thirty Bastis
  First one Anuvasana Basti is given, then alternately twelve Niruha and twelve Anuvasana are given, and finally five Anuvasana are given.
- Kala – Total course is sixteen Bastis
  First one Anuvasana, then alternately six Niruha and six Anuvasana are given, and finally three Anuvasana.
- Yoga – Total course of eight Bastis
  First one Anuvasana is given, then alternately three Anuvasana and three Niruha, and finally one Anuvasana.

Indications and Contraindications for Cleansing (Niruha) Enema

Cleansing enemas, those using less oil and more detoxifying herbs, are indicated in diseases of Vata due to obstruction in the channels. This consists mainly of pain conditions like pain in the abdomen, chest, pelvic region, eyes, ears or legs, headache, cardiac pain, hemiplegia, or facial paralysis. Usually Dashamula (the ten roots) decoction is the main ingredient in such enemas because it has a special power to remove Vata that is blocking the channels and causing pain.

Cleansing enemas are contraindicated in indigestion, obstruction or perforation in the intestines, for very old or debilitated patients, for toxins (Ama) in the gastrointestinal tract, diarrhea and vomiting. While not as potentially weakening to the patient as vomiting or purgation, it is still a depleting therapy and requires some caution in its application.

Indications and Contraindications for Oily (Anuvasana) Enema

Oily enemas have a more nutritive property than cleansing enemas. They are used for diseases of Vata due to tissue loss (wasting and debilitating diseases), like conditions of nervous exhaustion, sexual debility or just chronic low body weight. This method is contraindicated for persons with hemorrhoids, excessive Kapha in the gastrointestinal tract, low digestive power and ascites. The additional oil in the body can aggravate conditions of congestion and stagnation and weaken the digestive fire. But it is generally a safer procedure than the other methods because it is less potentially weakening to the patient.

Preparation of Cleansing Enemas

To prepare this type of enema, one must follow a sequence of mixing various ingredients. First add honey and rock salt, and mix them together in water. Then add the proper oleating material, like sesame oil or ghee, again mixing carefully. Then add a fine paste (Kalka) of herbs, and finally add it to the compound. The whole mixture, when thoroughly mixed, should be heated to body temperature. Then pour these contents into an enema bag. The quantity of the total mixture should range from 700 to 1200 cc. depending upon the age, disease and condition of the patient.

Procedure for Cleansing Enemas

This type of enema should be given four to six hours after eating, preferably early in the morning or in the evening. The patient should lie on a bed with the head low and in the left-lateral position. He should extend his left leg, with the right leg placed near the abdomen by folding it. He should keep his left hand below the head. A small amount of oil should be applied to the rectum as well as to the nozzle of the Basti applicator. The nozzle should be inserted slowly into the rectum. When all the contents of the Basti have entered into the large intestine, the nozzle should be slowly withdrawn. The medicated contents should be retained in the intestine for some time and then allowed to come out again along with the fecal matter and excess Pitta and Kapha. The patient should use a bedpan.

After treatment, the patient should take a rest. Then he is given warm water and, when hungry, should take a nutritive diet consisting of grains, milk and other rich substances.

Preparation of Oil Enemas

For this enema, medicated or plain sesame oil is used. The main procedure and post-enema treatment is the same as that of Niruha Basti. The only difference is that here, the quantity being small - from 60 to 100 cc. - a large plastic syringe can be used. The small quantity of the contents does not cause harm to the patient even when retained in the intestine for more than twenty-four hours. It is best to take this type of enema in the evening and to retain overnight if possible.

5. NASAL MEDICATION – Nasya

The nasal passages are the doorways to the mind and senses, the first site where Prana or vital energy is absorbed in the process of breathing. This Prana immediately nourishes the brain and senses and vitalizes the mind. Therefore, the right function of the nasal passages is necessary to keep our minds and senses clear and sharp. Nasya helps to clear the nasal channels by removing one of the main causes of disease, the toxins formed from wrong use of the mind and senses. Hence, this procedure is of great value for everyone and can be done safely on a regular basis.

In Nasya treatment, a medicated oil or powder is administered through the nose. In this way, the accumulated doshas above the region of clavicle in the head and neck are eliminated through the nose. This therapy is specifically advised for head, neck, ear, eye and throat diseases but can be an aid in treating many other types of diseases as well.

Types of Nasya

There are three ways of differentiating the various forms of nasal medications.

1. According to action

- Purification (Shodhana) or Purgation (Virechana) for the elimination of doshas
- Palliation (Shamana) for the reduction of doshas
- Tonifying (Brimhana) for subsidence of Vata

2. According to the substance used

- Avapida - Medicines put into the nose like herbal extracts
- Navana - Instilling liquids into the nose like milk and oils
- Dhuma - Inhaling the smoke of various herbs
- Virechana-Dhumapana - Applying medicinal powders into the nose with a special apparatus.

3. According to the dose

- Pratimarsha - A dose of only 2 drops in each nostril
- Marsha - 8 to 32 drops in each nostril.

Indications for Liquid Nasya (Avapida and Navana)

The main Nasya therapy is to apply drops of medicated oil into the nose. This is a Palliation type of Nasya indicated in all Vata-caused diseases of the head, ears, eyes and nose. It is also useful in Vata and Pitta-caused diseases of the mouth, falling out of hair, or dryness of the throat. Usually Anu Taila is used for this purpose, though simple sesame oil can be used as well. This mild type of Nasya can be done as part of health maintenance regimens, particularly for Vata people or in Vata climates and seasons when the nasal passages easily get dry and cause various problems of breathing and allergies. It is easy to do and can greatly improve how we feel and think. It is one of the simple, yet great healing methods of Ayurveda.

Indications for Dry Nasya (Dhuma and Dhumapana Nasya)

This type of Nasya uses powders or the smoke of various herbs. Dhumapana Nasya is a purificatory type of Nasya indicated in diseases where Kapha must be eliminated from the head region, as in sinusitis, heaviness in the head, epilepsy, or loss of voice. When a patient has too much congestion in the head for oil Nasya to work, this method should be employed to clear out the obstruction.

For this purpose, the powder of rock salt, garlic, dry ginger, calamus and black pepper is used and snuffed into the nose in the appropriate dosage. Simple calamus powder can also be used or even simple ginger powder, if these are the only herbs available. For Purification type of smoking therapy (Dhuma Nasya), guggul and other medicated resins are smoked.

Procedure for Nasya

After attending to his daily morning routine, the patient should clean his teeth and mouth. Then Pañchaguna or Bala oil is applied to his forehead and face and warm fomentation applied. Lastly, light massage is performed on the frontal part of the head, throat and cheeks. This oil application and massage serves to loosen the toxins in the head to assist in their removal.

Nasya of the liquid type is carried out when the patient is sitting or when lying on a bed. If the patient is lying in bed, then the head-end of the bed or table should be lowered a little. The patient should extend his neck so that his nostrils face upwards. Then medicated oil should be placed into the nostrils. Soon secretions begin to come from the nose. Afterwards, there is a sensation of lightness in the head and the disease symptoms are reduced. Nasya, if properly done, improves the functions of all the sense organs and makes one feel refreshed and awake.

After treatment, mild fomentation and massage should be applied over the forehead, cheeks and throat to soothe the patient. The patient should clear the throat of any residual amounts of the Nasya medication and gargle with hot water. Inhalation of medicated smoke, if available, may be done at this time. Nasya, using powders, can be done in a similar manner and has similar results.

THERAPEUTIC BLOOD-LETTING - Raktamosha

The great Ayurvedic doctor Sushruta includes both types of enemas in one category and regards bloodletting as the fifth procedure of Pancha Karma. Sushruta placed much importance on the blood, perhaps because he was a surgeon, considering it as the fourth Dosha in the body. Pure blood possesses a life-giving value, while impure blood creates and spreads diseases. Hence, impure blood should be removed from the body. Sushruta emphasizes this therapy just as Charaka emphasizes enemas (Basti).

Pitta dosha has a special affinity with the blood. When Pitta is aggravated and cannot be treated by the usual medicines, bloodletting can be very helpful. Hence, this is perhaps the most important therapy for diseases due to toxic blood and Pitta.

Bloodletting is indicated for diseases that are not amenable to hot and oily therapeutic measures (as most Vata diseases), hot and dry therapies (as most Kapha diseases), or to cold and dry measures (as most Pitta diseases). It is indicated for diseases due to simultaneous aggravation of blood and Pitta (a condition called Rakta-Pitta, or Pitta in the blood, in Sanskrit).

Types of Therapeutic Bloodletting

1. With sharp instruments:
   Prachhana - Making quick sharp incisions
   Siravyadha - Venesection
2. With blunt instruments (included here is the application of leeches)

Usually when blood and Pitta caused diseases are widespread, venesection (drawing blood from the veins) is used. When the disease is localized, leeches are used. Conditions treated by bloodletting include skin diseases like erysipelas, scabies, eczema, abscesses and vitiligo; inflammatory diseases like stomatitis, gingivitis and hemorrhoids; and liver diseases like jaundice and ascites.

This procedure is best carried out in October or just before the winter season. Venesection is performed with a simple syringe with a No. 18 needle or with the help of a bloodletting apparatus. An amount of 300 cc. of blood is taken from an adult patient. The patient should first be prepared with proper Oleation and Sudation as usual for all Pancha Karma procedures.

When leeches are used, the particular part of the body should be thoroughly washed with water (disinfectant drugs should not be applied to the skin). Then a scratch should be made or a drop of milk put on the skin where the leech will be placed. As soon as the leech starts sucking the blood, it should be covered with a damp gauze. After sucking sufficient blood, the leech automatically separates from the skin. The small wound made by the leech should be dressed with medicated oil and firmly bandaged.

Bloodletting is not used much in Ayurveda today. Sometimes Ayurvedic doctors recommend that Pitta types donate blood instead in order to deal with their tendency to produce excess or toxic blood. Other times they recommend strong alterative (blood-cleansing) herbs like turmeric, manjishta or neem. Bloodletting is still sometimes used in Chinese medicine, and is usually performed on the patient's back.

11 Marma Points: Ayurvedic Pressure Points

Marma means secret, hidden, vital energy. Marmas are special points of energy and vulnerability located throughout the entire body. Each marma is a receptor point on the skin that relates to different bodily organs and tissues, and through which vital energy currents pass. They are the points through which Prana, the master energy and intelligence of our psychophysical system, travels and through which it can be directed.

Marma points are much like the acupuncture points of Traditional Chinese Medicine. One finds the first reference to them in the *Atharva Veda*. Sushruta deals with them elaborately. Knowledge of these sensitive anatomical points was applied in war for harming the enemy or for protecting oneself. This knowledge became an essential part of training for surgeons, as injury to these points can produce death or disability.

A Marma point is defined as an anatomical site where flesh, veins, arteries, tendons, bones and joints meet. As the technique of massage developed, these points were used for stimulating internal organs and systems of the body. Marma points are classified according to the different areas on the body where they occur, the tissue of which they are composed, and the effects which are felt if they are injured.

Like the Chinese acupuncture points, Marma points are measured by the finger units (Anguli) relative to each individual. Their size is measured by finger inches, and their location determined by them. However, the Marma points differ from acupuncture points in that a number of Marmas are larger in size and mark areas from one to eight finger units in diameter. As indicating a larger area, rather than a point, their definition is general.

Number of Marma Points

By Region of the Body

Upper Limbs – 22	Lower Limbs – 22	Abdomen & Thorax – 12
Back & Trunk – 14	Head & Neck – 37	

By Structure

Muscular – 11	Blood Vessels – 41	Ligaments & Tendons – 27
Joints – 20	Bone – 8	

By Signs (if injured)

1) Causing instant death (Sadyaha Pranahara) – 9
2) Causing death in time (Kalantara Pranahara) – 33
3) Causing death if hit by a foreign body like a bullet (Vishalyaghnakara) – 3
4) Painful (Rujakara) – 8
5) Causing disability (Vikalatvakara) – 44

Explanation of Sanskrit Marma Names

Most of the Marmas are named after their location or function. Hence, their name helps to identify them. Many of these points can be treated either at the front or at the back of the body part that relates to them.

HANDS & LEGS

Talahridaya—heart or center of the palm of the hand or sole of the foot
Kshipra—quick, owing to its immediate effects
Kurccha—a knot or bundle of muscles or tendons at the base of the thumb or big toe
Kurcchashira—the head of kurccha, at the base of the hand or the foot
Manibanda—bracelet, as it goes around wrist
Gulpha—ankle joint
Indrabasti—Indra's bladder, mid-forearm and mid-calf
Kurpara—elbow joint
Janu—knee joint
Ani—the lower region of the upper arm or leg
Urvi—the wide, the wide mid-region of the thigh or forearm
Lohitaksha—red eyed, the lower frontal insert of the shoulder joint and leg joint
Kakshadhara—what upholds the flanks, the top of the Shoulder joint
Vitapa—the perineum, where the legs are connected to the trunk

ABDOMEN

Guda—anus
Basti—bladder
Nabhi—navel

THORAX

Hridaya—heart
Stanamula—root of the breast
Stanarohita—incline (or upper region) of the breast
Apastambha—a point on the upper side of the chest said to carry the Prana or life-force
Apalapa—unguarded, the armpit or axilla

BACK

Kukundara—marking the loins, on either side of the posterior superior iliac spine
Katikataruna—what arises from the sacrum, the center of the buttocks
Nitamba—the upper region of the buttocks
Parshwasandhi—the joint of the sides, the side of the waist
Brihati—the large or broad region of the back
Amshaphalaka—the shoulderblade
Amsa—the shoulder

NECK

Manya—honor, perhaps owing to its connection with the voice
Nila—dark blue, from the color of the veins at this point
Sira Matrika—the mother of the blood vessels" from the arteries to the head that flow through this region
Krikatika—the joint of the neck

HEAD

Vidhura—distress, from its sensitive nature
Phana—a serpent's hood, the side of the nostrils
Apanga—the outer corner of the eye
Avarta—calamity, from its sensitive nature
Shankha—conch, the temple
Utkshepa—what is thrown upwards, as it is above the temple
Sthapani—what gives support
Shringatakani—places where four roads meet, the soft palate of the mouth
Simanta—the summit, the skull and surrounding joints
Adhipati—the overlord

TABLE OF MARMA POINTS

Name and Extent Finger Unit	#	Site	Location	Composition	Effects of severe injury	Importance in treatment

HANDS AND LEGS

Name and Extent Finger Unit	#	Site	Location	Composition	Effects of severe injury	Importance in treatment
Talahridaya 1/2 Anguli	4	Both palms & soles	Center of palm & sole	Muscular	Slow death	Stimulation of Lung
Kshipra 1/2 Anguli	4	Both hands & feet	Between thumb & index finger and first and second toes	Tendon	Slow death	Stimulation of Heart
Kurccha 4 Anguli	4	Both palms & soles	2 Anguli above Kshipra Marma, root of thumb	Tendon	Disability, pain, tremors	Kurccha Marma on sole controls Alochaka Pitta

Name and Extent Finger Unit	#	Site	Location	Composition	Effects of severe injury	Importance in treatment
			HANDS AND LEGS (cont'd)			
Kurcchashira 1 Anguli	4	Both palms & feet	1) Just below wrist joint 2) At center of the heel below Gulpha Marma	Tendon	Pain	
Manibanda 2 Anguli	2	Both hands	Wrist joint	Joint	Pain	
Gulpha 2 Anguli	2	Both legs	Ankle joint	Joint	Pain	
Indrabasti 1/2 Anguli	4	Both mid-fore-arm & mid-calf regions	In the center of area	Muscu-lar	Anemia, slow death	Stimulation of Agni (di-gestive fire) and small intestine
Kurpara 3 Anguli	2	Both hands	Elbow joint	Joint	Disability	Stimulation of Liver and Spleen
Ani 1/2 Anguli	4	Arms & thighs	3 Anguli above Kurpara and Janu	Tendon	Disability and swel-ling on the thigh	
Urvi 1 Anguli	4	Upper arm & thigh	Middle of upper arm or thigh	Blood vessel	Atrophy of thigh muscles, anemia	Stimulation of Ambhu-vaha Srotas
Lohitaksha 1/2 Anguli	4	Armpit & in-guinal region	Joint of groin or shoulders	Blood vesel	Disability, paralysis due to blood loss	
Kakshadhara 1 Anguli	2	Front arm	2 Anguli above Lohita-ksha	Liga-ment of shoul-der joint	Disability	
Vitapa 1 Anguli	2	Front of the ab-domen	2 Anguli be-low Lohitak-sha, at root of scrotum	Inguinal	Disability, importence	

Name and Extent Finger Unit	#	Site	Location	Composition	Effects of severe injury	Importance in treatment

ABDOMEN

Name and Extent Finger Unit	#	Site	Location	Composition	Effects of severe injury	Importance in treatment
Guda Anguli	1	Around anus		Muscular	Sudden death	Stimulation of 4 first chakra, re-productive & urinary systems
Basti 4 Anguli	1	Ab-domen	In between pubic sym-physis & umbilicus	Ligament	Sudden death	Control of Kapha
Nabhi 4 Anguli	1	Ab-domen	Around umbilicus	Ligament	Sudden death	Control of small intes-tine and Pachaka Pitta

THORAX

Name and Extent Finger Unit	#	Site	Location	Composition	Effects of severe injury	Importance in treatment
Hridaya 4 Anguli	1	Chest	Middle of sternum	Blood vessel	Sudden death	Control of Sadhaka Pitta, Vyana Vayu
Stanamula 2 Anguli	2	Chest	Below the nipple	Blood vessel	Slow death	
Stanarohita 1/2 Anguli	2	Chest	2 Anguli above Stanamula	Muscular	Slow death	
Apastambha 1/2 Anguli	2	Chest	In midline bet. nipple & collar bone	Blood vessel	Slow death	
Apalapa 1/2 Anguli	2	Chest	Lateral side of Stanarohita	Blood vessel	Slow death	

Name and Extent Finger Unit	#	Site	Location	Composition	Effects of severe injury	Importance in treatment
			BACK			
Katikataruna 1/2 Anguli	2	On buttocks	Center of hip	Bone	Slow death	Control of adipose tissue
Kukundara 1/2 Anguli	2	Back	On each post. sup. iliac spine	Joint	Disability	Control of second chakra
Nitamba 1/2 Anguli	2	Back	4 Anguli above & lateral to Kukundara	Bone	Slow death	
Parshwasandhi 1/2 Anguli		Back	2 Anguli above Nitamba	Blood vessel	Slow death	
Brihati 1/2 Anguli	2	Back	2 Anguli below lateral side of spine	Blood vessel	Slow death	Control of third chakra
Amsaphalaka 1/2 Anguli	2	Back	On scapula bone above Brihati	Bone	Disability, atrophy of shoulder muscles	Control of fourth chakra
Amsa 1/2 Anguli	2	Back	4 Anguli above Amsaphalaka, between shoulder and neck		Ligament Disability, frozen shoulder	Control of fifth chakra
			NECK			
Manya 4 Anguli	2	Neck	Posterior side of larynx	Blood vessel	Disability	Control of blood
Nila 4 Anguli	2	Neck	Anterior side of larynx	Blood vessel	Disability	
Sira Matrika 4 Anguli	8	Neck	Four arteries on each side of neck	Blood vessel	Sudden death	
Krikatika /2 Anguli	2	Neck	Junction of head and neck	Joint	Disability	

Name and Extent Finger Unit	#	Site	Location	Composition	Effects of severe injury	Importance in treatment
			HEAD			
Vidhura 1/2 Anguli	2	Neck	Below both ears	Tendon	Disability, deafness	
Phana 1/2 Anguli	2	Face	On both sides of nostrils	Blood vessels	Disabil- ity, loss of smell	
Apanga 1/2 Anguli	2	Face	Lateral corner of eyes	Blood vessels	Disability, blindness	
Avarta 1/2 Anguli	2	Face	Above eyebrows on lateral side	Joint	Disability, Blindness	
Shankha 2 Anguli	2	Head	Temple, between ear and Apanga	Bone	Sudden death	Control of large intestine
Utkshepa 1/2 Anguli	2	Head	Above Shankha Marma	Ligament	Vishal- yaghna (Death occurs if foreign body is removed)	Control of large intestine
Sthapani 1/2 Anguli	1	Head	In between the center of eyebrows	Blood vessel	Vishal- yaghna	Control of mind and nerves by oil appli- cation
Shringa- takani 4 Anguli	4	Head	Soft palate	Blood	Sudden death	Control of nerves
Simanta Linear	5	Head	On the joints of skull bones	Joint	Slow death	Control of nerves
Adhipati 1/2 Anguli	1	Head	Center of occiput	Joint	Sudden death	Control of mind and nerves

Effects of Particular Marma Points (note drawings 241-242)

KANTHA (Throat): Connected to the vocal cords and to the tonsils. If there is hoarseness of voice or laryngitis, this point becomes very sensitive.

SVARA: Thyroid cartilage. The thyroid is the gland of Agni, or the bodily fire, which controls metabolism.

JATRU: River of Prana. Connected to the Bronchi and the Trachea. Pressing this point can relieve Bronchial Asthma and wheezing. Helps dilation of Bronchi and Trachea if gently pressed. Connects to the lungs.

AKSHAK: The right side point relates to gall bladder, the left side to the spleen.

STHAPANI (Third Eye): Used for awakening Kundalini. Connected to pituitary gland. Gives will power, harmony, order, judgement, balance and command.

KANINIKA: Connected to the liver. Can be very sensitive. The pulse can be felt at this point. Chanting "Ram" stimulates the liver from this point.

NASA AGRA: Connected to the heart. If pressed, helps to dilate bronchi.

OSHTA: Dilates mid-cerebral artery, stops convulsions immediately. Prevents fainting or vertigo.

HANU: Helps release tension in the heart. Allows for inner surrender. Connect to the seed mantra "Yam" for the heart.

SHANKHA: Tenderness of this point indicates migraine headaches, dizziness or TMJ problems.

KSHIPRA: Related to the colon and emotions. Pressure here on the right side point relieves anger, on the left side point relieves fear. Tenderness indicates toxins in the colon and low energy.

Stimulation of Marma Points

Marmas are most easily stimulated by pressure applied with

the fingers, particularly with the thumb. Press deeply but not painfully and hold the pressure for one to three minutes. This should be followed by gentle massage of the region. It can be done along with body massage therapy. Points on the head are most sensitive and should be done with some gentleness. Points on the back are harder to reach. Points on the abdomen are also very sensitive. Points on the arms and legs, particularly

MARMANI (energy points)

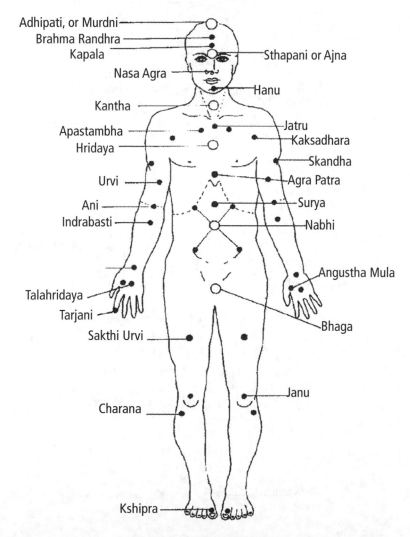

Adhipati, or Murdni
Brahma Randhra
Kapala
Nasa Agra
Sthapani or Ajna
Hanu
Kantha
Jatru
Apastambha
Kaksadhara
Hridaya
Skandha
Urvi
Agra Patra
Ani
Surya
Indrabasti
Nabhi
Angustha Mula
Talahridaya
Tarjani
Bhaga
Sakthi Urvi
Janu
Charana
Kshipra

the hands and feet, are the easiest to work on and are very powerful in their effects.

Another method is to apply a stimulating oil to the site, like camphor or eucalyptus, which can be left on and then washed off during the patient's next shower.

MARMANI (energy points)

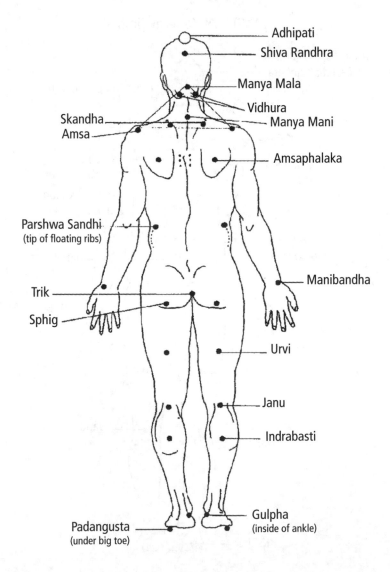

12 Treatment of the Channel Systems (Srotamsi)

The human body consists of a marvelous and elaborate network of channels connecting all the organs and tissues together, supplying them with nutrients and removing their waste-materials. Ayurveda recognizes fourteen such channel-systems that approximate the physiological systems of modern medicine and govern all bodily functions. In Sanskrit these channels are called *srotas* in the singular, or *srotamsi* in the plural, which literally means a channel or a current. They are different from the nadis or channels of the subtle body which exist at a deeper level, and are also different from acupuncture meridians, which are also subtler. But these physical channels connect with those more subtle, including those of Prana and the mind, which have their own channel systems.

Health consists of the right flow of energy and nutrition through these channels, supplying and cleansing the tissues and organs of the body. Disease occurs when proper flow is somehow impaired or obstructed. Ayurvedic diagnosis and treatment follows the channel systems (Srotas) because these cover all the functions of the body (and mind). It examines which channels are affected by disease, in what manner and to what degree. The channels provide a means of gauging not only the nature but also the level of the disease. The following chapter outlines these different systems, their dysfunctions

243

and their typical treatment methods.

THE FOURTEEN CHANNEL SYSTEMS

Three Channels Bring in Nourishment

1. PRANAVAHA SROTAS: The channels that carry Prana, the breath or life-force.
2. AMBHUVAHA SROTAS: The channels that carry water (ambhu) or regulate water metabolism.
3. ANNAVAHA SROTAS: The channels that carry food (anna). Mainly the digestive system.

Seven Channels Supply the Seven Tissues of the Body

4. RASAVAHA SROTAS: The channels that carry plasma (rasa).
5. RAKTAVAHA SROTAS: The channels that carry blood (rakta).
6. MAMSAVAHA SROTAS: The channels that supply the muscles (mamsa).
7. MEDOVAHA SROTAS: The channels that supply fat or adipose tissue (medas).
8. ASTHIVAHA SROTAS: The channels that supply the bones (asthi) or the skeletal system.
9. MAJJAVAHA SROTAS: The channels that supply the marrow and nerve tissue (majja), mainly the nervous system (cerebrospinal fluid).
10. SHUKRAVAHA SROTAS: The channels that supply the reproductive tissue (shukra) or the reproductive system.

Two special subsystems of the reproductive system exist within the female for purposes of reproduction:

ARTAVAVAHA SROTAS: The channels that carry menstruation (artava).

STANYAVAHA SROTAS: The channels that carry the breast milk (stanya).

Three Channels Allow for Elimination

11. MUTRAVAHA SROTAS: The channels that carry urine (mutra) or the urinary system.

12. PURISHAVAHA SROTAS: The channels that carry feces (purisha) or the excretory system.

13. SWEDAVAHA SROTAS: The channels that carry sweat (sweda) or the sebaceous system.

The Mind Exists as a Special Channel System

14. MANOVAHA SROTAS: The channels that carry thought or the mental system.

Health is the proper flow through these channels. When unobstructed, they supply nutrients and remove waste materials, and also serve to maintain communication between the different tissues and organs. Disease is nothing but improper flow through the channels.

The Four Improper Flows Through the Channels

1. Excessive flow	2. Deficient flow
3. Blockage of flow	4. Flow outside of the proper channel

- Excessive flow occurs when the flow through the channels is too much or too quick. This floods the tissues and they can hyperfunction or become overly developed.
- Deficient flow is when the flow is too light or too slow. This causes the tissues to hypofunction, to dry up or accumulate waste materials.
- Blockage of flow occurs when the Doshas, waste materials or Ama accumulate, stagnate and harden in the channels. This also blocks the supply to the tissues, which causes them to accumulate waste materials and deprives them of nutrition.
- Flow outside of the proper channel usually is a result of blockage of flow. What is not allowed to flow in the normal way, like water, will try to flow in an abnormal way. This

will cause a flow of improper substances into tissues or may break the channels and directly invade the tissues.

Usually, improper flow is caused by some excess or inappropriate material accumulating in the channels which causes pain. The excess Doshas (mainly Kapha and Pitta), toxins (Ama) and waste-materials move into the channels causing these various types of improper flow. Vata (wind), as governing all impulses and energy flow, is the main factor regulating the flow in the channels. Its dryness can also block the channels. Clearing the channels is an important concept in Ayurvedic healing.

TREATMENT THROUGH THE CHANNEL SYSTEMS

Respiratory System – Pranavaha Srotas

Diseases

Prana, or the life-force, is the key energy in the body. In fact, the physical body is enveloped, energized and sustained by a pranic body or pranic field around it. The pranic channel system, therefore, is the most important of the channel systems and serves to energize them all. Its origin is in the heart and the gastro-intestinal tract. The combined heart and lung apparatus is the main seat of this system. Although it can be equated with the respiratory system, Pranavaha srotas is much more than that. Its action extends to the brain and its centers, which is the chief site of the life-force or Prana. It also connects to the large intestine where prana from the food is absorbed.

Causes of disturbance to this system are malnutrition, wasting diseases, excessive physical exercise, dehydration, polluted air and dust, as well as an excess of Vata or Kapha. Trauma and injury effect this system quickly as well. Signs of imbalance are rapid, shallow, abnormal, disturbed, or painful respiration. Additional symptoms are cough, wheezing, discoloration due to dyspnea, and various inflammatory conditions of the lungs and upper respiratory tract.

Treatment

Treatment is mainly according to the treatment of asthma. One should consider the prominence of Vata and Kapha in general; for inflammatory conditions of the lungs, Pitta must be treated as well. Typical herbs are vasa, licorice, horehound, elecampane and ephedra. Aromatic oils like eucalyptus or camphor are important for opening the lungs and stimulating the flow of prana and can be massaged externally into the chest.

Sthapani Marma, the point that lies between the eyebrows, and Talahridaya Marmas, the point at the center of both the palms of the hand and soles of feet, should be massaged with warm oils to stimulate the lungs and heart. In particular, Dhara Tail should be applied on Sthapani Marma.

Pranayama is naturally a key therapy. Alternate nostril breathing should be done regularly to increase the strength of the heart-lung system. As the mind is related to Vata, when respiratory diseases arise due to disturbed thoughts and emotions, the practice of meditation is essential. As the heart, on an energetic level, is part of this system, developing deeper feelings and greater connections with others is helpful.

Water Metabolism System – Ambhuvaha Srotas

Diseases

The palate and the pancreas are the origins of this system that governs the absorption of water in the body. It is damaged by excesses of alcohol and other liquids, by not taking proper fluids, by eating too many dry food substances, by working in the heat, by fright, and by indigestion. Excess salt intake and inadequate intake of fluids are additional factors. Signs of its imbalances are dryness of the mouth, constant thirst, retention of fluid in various organs as in pleurisy, ascites, the formation of tumors with fluid inside, and generalized edema. Diabetes is the most characteristic disease of this system.

Treatment

This system is treated along the line of treatment for excessive thirst (trishna). In these diseases, reducing Vata is the key, while increasing the intake of fluids, oils and tonic herbs like shatavari or amalaki, particularly by taking sour liquids, sugar and salt, the Kapha-increasing tastes.

If too much fluid has accumulated in any organ or if there is edema, which are mainly Kapha conditions, then salt restriction and potassium supplementation should occur. Diuretic herbs like punarnava, gokshura, and lemon grass are important in this case. For diabetes, herbs like turmeric, guggul, shilajit and gurmar are helpful, as well as bitters like neem and aloe.

Treating Basti Marma, the point between the umbilicus and pubic region which controls Kapha, is important, as water is the chief element of Kapha. Along with this, treating Urvi Marma in the mid-upper arm and mid-thigh region gives excellent results.

Digestive System – Annavaha Srotas

Diseases

The esophagus and stomach are the chief seats of this system. Its origin is in the stomach and the left side of the body. It is damaged by eating junk food, fast food, improper food, food that is not properly cooked or is overcooked, unwholesome food having an improper mixture of substances, bad food combinations as well as by any irregular eating habits. Signs of its impairment are indigestion, gas formation, pain or burning sensation in the gastric region, nausea, vomiting, and on rare occasions, vomiting with blood.

Treatment

Most disorders of the digestive system originate due to disturbances in Jatharagni, or the digestive fire. Hence, correction of the digestive fire is the key to treating the diseases of this system. Herbs like Trikatu (ginger, black pepper, and long pepper), chitrak and cayenne are good for this purpose. High Pitta conditions like hyperacidity and ulcers should be treated with demulcent herbs like shatavari, amalaki, and licorice, and bland food like milk and mung beans. For Vata type nervous digestion, asafoetida, garlic and mineral salts are good.

For stimulating digestion through Marma points, the four Indra Basti Marmas, two on the mid-lower arm and two at the mid-calf region, should be used. These points can be massaged with medicated oils containing hot herbs like ginger and cinnamon.

Circulatory System, Plasma or Lymph Portion – Rasavaha Srotas

Diseases

The heart and blood vessels are the origins of this system. Through this system, the absorbed portion of food circulates along with the lymph and blood and supplies nutrients to the tissues. Hence, if food is not digested properly owing to a low digestive fire, thereby creating Ama, this system gets disturbed, carrying toxins rather than the proper nutrition. Excess eating and drinking and too much stress and strain are other aggravating factors. All the abnormalities of the SA node in the heart, which disturb circulation, and other heart conditions, including enlargement of the heart, damage it as well.

Signs of its imbalance are disinclination for food, anorexia, bad taste in the mouth, impotence, wasting away of the body tissues, weakening of the digestive fire, premature formation of wrinkles, and premature graying of the hair. Along with these signs, palpitations, bradycardia, tachycardia, or angina should be present as well. Remember the connection of plasma or rasa with the skin; abnormalities of the skin reflect problems with the plasma.

Treatment

While treating the plasma system, proper attention must be given to maintaining its optimal circulation in the body. In Naturopathy, a special kind of massage is used to improve the circulation of lymph, called "lymph drainage massage." On the front of the body, one should massage the neck down to the clavicle and sternum. As the armpits and groin contain many lymph nodes, proper attention must also be paid to these areas, and the abdomen as well, using circular strokes.

As the lymph is Kapha in nature, a general anti-Kapha therapy preventing mucus formation is indicated, with the use of sweating agents like ginger, cinnamon or sage and expectorants like bayberry or elecampane. Saunas and steam baths are also helpful. The digestive fire should be maintained in good order as described under Annavaha Srotas.

When Vata is involved, as with low body fluids and dry skin, oil massage is necessary using medicated sesame oils and tonic herbs that build the plasma like shatavari, marshmallow or rehmannia. Dairy products are helpful, particularly milk, which itself is a form of plasma.

Circulatory System, Blood or Hemoglobin Portion – Raktavaha Srotas

Diseases

The liver and spleen are the origins of this system as they are responsible for the formation of the blood. Causes that impair this system are mainly those of high Pitta because the blood is connected with Pitta. Food that is very spicy or hot and causes a burning sensation will overheat the blood. Excessively oily or greasy food can damage the blood, as can too much salt or acidic food. Injury is another factor. Any excess bleeding naturally weakens the blood, including excess menstrual bleeding in women. Psychological factors are stress, overwork and other Pitta increasing emotional factors, like anger and irritability.

Signs of impairment are skin disorders like acne and skin rashes, blood in the urine or feces, bleeding under the skin, inflammation of the rectum, and stomatitis. Anemia, enlargement of liver and spleen, abscesses, tumors, bluish-black spots on the skin, jaundice and leucoderma are additional factors.

Treatment

Palliation of Pitta and the use of alterative or blood-cleansing herbs like manjishta, turmeric, red clover or burdock are the most important part of the treatment. Ayurvedic coral oxide (Prawal Bhasma) and pearl oxide (Moti Bhasma), and bitter purgatives like rhubarb root are helpful to cool the blood. When conditions like anemia exist, diet and herbs to increase the blood like green vegetables and Suvarna Makshika (a purified iron compound) should be given, along with tonic herbs like amalaki, dan gui or turmeric.

For stimulating the blood system, massage to certain Marma points is a must, especially Hridaya Marma. The twelve Marma points in the region of the throat, the eight Sira Matruka Marmas on both sides of the neck, the two Nila, and two Manya Marmas should also be considered.

Muscular System – Mamsavaha Srotas

Diseases

The ligaments and skin are the main origins of this system. It is imbalanced by over-consumption of heavy, oily and greasy food, by sleeping after eating and by improper exercise. Kapha is the main dosha connected to it. All diseases arising out of the muscles like various tumors, piles, warts, sloughing of flesh, and gangrene in the muscle, are signs of its impairment. Muscular pain is generally due to high Vata and muscular inflammation due to high Pitta.

Treatment

For treating muscular pain, rubefacient herbs that increase blood circulation and remove pain like mustard and cinnamon should be used if the pain is due to injury and congestion. If the pain is due to high Vata, then anti-Vata tonifying herbs like shatavari and oils prepared from it like Narayan oil should be used. If the pain is due to Vata that is increased due to ob-struction, then oils like Vishgarbha should be used, along with anti-spasmodic herbs like jatamamsi and valerian.

For treating muscle tumors, the digestive fire of the muscle tissue (Mamsavaha Agni) should be improved by using herbs like ashwagandha. If it is not possible to eliminate muscle tumors by these means, then Agnikarma, cauterization by using probes of gold, copper or iron, or cauterization by alkalies prepared out of plants should be used. In severe cases, surgery may be required.

Adipose System – Medovaha Srotas

Diseases

The fat around the kidneys and abdominal fat are the origins of this system. Excessive consumption of fatty substances, too much eating of sweet, salty and sour foods, dairy products, sugar, beef and meat imbalance this system. Lack of exercise and over-indulgence in wine are other factors. Obesity and diseases arising out of obesity like hypertension, heart disease, diabetes, and arthritis are the chief diseases of this system. Lipomas or fatty tumors and conditions of arteriosclerosis are also important disease conditions.

Treatment

The main factor in treating this system is to normalize the metabolism of the adipose tissue. For this, fat-reducing herbs like guggul, myrrh and rasna should be used in combinations with those like cyperus, chitrak, or black pepper which stimulate digestion and burning up of fat. Bitters like aloe or gentian, which have a reducing effect, are also good. Deep massage work with dry powders of talcum or calamus, or with hot oils like mustard, is another good practice.

Kapha is closely linked with adipose tissue. Hence, it is good to give Vamana or herb-induced emesis and other anti-Kapha therapies. Sweating therapy (swedana) is excellent, either through herbs like ginger and cinnamon or through heat induced saunas. Anti-Kapha diet and increased exercise is also important, as is reducing the amount of sleep.

In obese patients, Guda Marma should be massaged. If this is tender, then it should be considered as an indication of some obstruction in the system. At such times therapeutic vomiting is helpful to get rid of excess Kapha obstructing the channels.

Skeletal System – Asthivaha Srotas

Diseases

Adipose tissue and the bones of the hips are the origins of this system. The bones and Vata are closely related. This means that if the colon, the chief site of Vata, gets disturbed, or if Vata otherwise becomes imbalanced, then this system will also have problems. Similarly, external injuries causing fractures, violent movements of the body, and a Vata-increasing diet can damage this system. Pain in the bones, hypertrophy or atrophy of bones, discoloration and other pathological conditions of the hair and nails, and various tumors of the bones indicate diseases of this system. Arthritis is the main chronic disorder.

Treatment

Substances that contain natural calcium, like oyster shells or sesame seeds, help build the bones. Enemas with sesame oil or those containing milk, ghee and nutritive herbs like ashwagandha and shatavari are extremely good as well. These herbs are also good taken as food supplements. Red coral powder (prawal) is excellent. Anti-arthritic and analgesic herbs like nirgundi, guggul, angelica and cayenne are important. Triphala is excellent for regulating Vata in the colon and thereby protecting the bones.

Vata should be controlled by stimulating Sthapani and Adhipati Marmas. For correcting disturbances in the colon, Shankha Marma in the temples and Utkshepa Marma just below it should be massaged.

Nervous System – Majjavaha Srotas

Diseases

The long bones and joints, which house the nerve tissue and bone marrow, are the origins of this system. The main causes of its dysfunction are injuries to the skull, vertebral column and other long bones, which crush the marrow. Infections, high fevers, and improper food habits that increase Vata also disturb this system. Pain in the joints, giddiness, fainting, lack of coordination in movement, tremors, paralysis or paresis of the muscles, and wrong reception of sensations of touch and temperature are important signs of its diseases. Typical diseases range from insomnia to various nervous disorders.

Treatment

Both high Vata and high Pitta disturb this system. As Pitta's site of accumulation is the small intestine, through controlling this organ, one can also control excess Pitta in the nervous system. Nervine stimulants like calamus, shankha pushpi and pippali, as well as sedatives like gotu kola, jatamamsi, valerian and shankhapushpi are primary. Many tonics like ashwagandha also have nutritive properties for the nerves. Nuts, like almonds and walnuts, and oils, like ghee and sesame, nourish the nerves.

The five Simanta Marmas situated in the cranial sutures and the four Sringataka Marmas should be treated appropriately. Sthapani and Adhipati Marmas treated by Shirodhara (dripping of medicated oil) is good for disorders like insomnia, loss of sensory function and paralysis. Enema treatment with tonifying oils like sesame are excellent.

Reproductive System – Shukravaha Srotas

Diseases

In men, the testes and penis are the chief sites of this system (for women see the Menstrual System). Untimely sexual intercourse or unnatural sexual acts, excessive sexual indulgence, suppression of the sexual urge, and bad effects of various surgical procedures lie behind the various diseases of this system. These deplete Ojas and increase Vata, which causes Vata disorders like tuberculosis, consumption, or other wasting disorders (including AIDS). Permanent sterility or impotency can result. Diseases like enlargement of the prostate and hydrocele are included here.

Treatment

In cases of sexual debility, food and herbs that increase the reproductive fluids are indicated like dairy products, nuts, eggs and shellfish. Rejuvenative (Rasayana) and invigorating (Vajikarana) herbs play an important part, like ashwagandha, shilajit, bala and shatavari. Kapikacchu is the best single herb.

Control of Apana Vayu is essential. For this, Guda Marma and Kukundara Marma should be treated with oil massage. Sexual abstinence can help rebuild this system, though sexual repression can block its flow.

Menstrual System – Artavavaha Srotas

Diseases

The uterus and fallopian tubes are the origins of this system, which governs female reproductive function. Increase of Pitta and Vata primarily cause its dysfunctions such as PMS, discomfort and pain during menstruation (dysmenorrhea), absence of menstruation (amenorrhea), excessive bleeding during menstruation (menorrhagia), and various disturbances at the time of menopause. The same sexual imbalances as can damage Shukravaha Srotas come into play here as well.

Treatment

In treating this system, Apana Vayu, the downward moving air, is most important. Hence, the same Marma points for the treatment of the urinary system should be considered.

Emmenagogue (menstruation-promoting) herbs like saffron, turmeric, pennyroyal or motherwort should be used as needed. For symptoms due to stress and strain or cramping pain, sedatives like valerian or jatamamsi should be added. Tonics like shatavari or dan gui nourish this system. Aloe gel is also good for Pitta problems here including night sweats and hot flashes, like those of menopause.

Lactation System – Stanyavaha Srotas

Diseases

The breasts and nipples are the origins of this system, which is active during the period of lactation after childbirth. Improper care of the breasts during pregnancy and food that increases

Vata and Kapha disturbs this system. Signs of its impairment are deficient milk supply, impure milk, breast tumors, or abscesses.

Treatment

For increasing the quantity of milk, galactagogue herbs like shatavari, licorice and sesame seeds are good, as well as a diet for increasing Kapha. For removing the bad qualities of milk due to excess doshas, cyperus, fennel, dill, or dandelion are good. For stopping the flow of the breast milk, sage is good taken cold.

Urinary System – Mutravaha Srotas

Diseases

The large intestine and urinary bladder are the origins of this system. It is damaged by excessive or insufficient drinking of water, by excessive heat and dry climate, by constantly working near fire, or exposure to toxic substances. Signs of its damage are painful urination, burning urination, lack of urination, urinary tract infections, or stones in the urinary system.

Treatment

Treatment is mainly through diuretic (urination promoting) herbs, of which there are many Western herbs such as corn silk, uva ursi or pippsessewa. Most frequently used in Ayurveda are punarnava and gokshura, which together balance the kidney energy. In inflammatory conditions, anti-Pitta herbs should be used like katuka, golden seal, or uva ursi. Demulcents like marshmallow and shatavari help with burning or difficult urination, particularly as associated with thirst, fever or dryness.

Katika, Taruna and Kukundar Marma, along with Basti Marma points, should be massaged. This stimulates the urinary organs in a beneficial manner.

Excretory System – Purishavaha Srotas

Diseases

The rectum and anal canal are the origins of this system. It is damaged by suppression of the urge to defecate, by eating food that has too much or too little roughage, or by lack of proper oil in the food. When the digestive power is weak, this system also gets disturbed along with it. Signs of its improper functioning are diarrhea, constipation, dysentery, pain in the colon, colitis, blood in the stool, and hemorrhoids.

Treatment

Treatment varies according to the condition. In cases of diarrhea, before giving astringent herbs to bind the stool, make sure that any toxins in the colon have first been flushed out with laxatives. Then one can use astringents like kutaj or alum. In amoebic dysentery, excess Kapha should be treated along with high Vata by giving sesame oil enemas. The herbal formula Triphala is good for mild constipation, while for severe constipation purgatives like castor oil, rhubarb root or senna leaf work better. Psyllium helps when one needs more bulk in the stool. Krikatika and Sandhi Marma are important points to massage for this system.

Sweating System – Swedavaha Srotas

Diseases

The origin of this system is in the adipose tissue and the pores on the skin. It is damaged by exposure to the elements (wind, cold, or heat) and by excessive exercise. Anger or fear, eating of hot and spicy food, excess or insufficient drinking of water, and drinking of wine are additional vitiating factors. Signs of its impairment are excess sweating, deficient sweating, skin rashes, or skin diseases.

Treatment

Treatment is mainly through diaphoretic (sweat-promoting)

herbs and through Oleation (Snehana) and Sudation (Swedana) therapies. Diaphoretic herbs like cinnamon, sage and ginger increase sweating while astringents like lodhra or alum root counter excess sweating. Aromatic oils like eucalyptus or camphor open up circulation in this system, while heavy oils like sesame help close it. Saunas and hot tubs stimulate it by promoting sweating through heat. Exercise also helps cleanse this system.

Mind – Manovaha Srotas

Diseases

The origin of this system is in the heart and in the nerve tissue. It is damaged by overwork, stress, worry, anxiety, fright, anger or grief. Physical factors are injury to the head, insomnia, taking of drugs, or derangements of the senses. Signs of its impairment are dizziness, distress, palpitations, emotional excesses or mental disorders.

Treatment

Owing to the mind's connection with Vata, most treatment will aim at reducing high Vata and calming its resultant agitation and instability. Treatment is mainly through herbs to calm and balance the mind like gotu kola (brahmi), calamus, shankha pushpi, jatamamsi and valerian. In cases of brain fatigue, tonics like ashwagandha and shatavari are also useful. Warm sesame oil massage to the head, including dripping the oil on the forehead (shirodhara) is excellent for calming Vata in the mind. Meditation is another important therapy. Stimulating the marmas in the head, particularly those at the top of the head, is also important.

13 *Yoga and Ayurveda*

A person who studies only one branch of learning cannot arrive at truth. Therefore, a physician should strive to learn as many related sciences as possible.
—*Sushruta*

Yoga has become popular worldwide as a physical health system emphasizing Yoga postures to improve the strength and flexibility of the body and to relieve stress. It also includes an entire system of meditation aimed at Self-realization. Ayurveda is similarly gaining recognition throughout the world as an important system of natural healing for the body and the mind. Yet many people do not understand how closely related Yoga and Ayurveda are and how usefully they work together.

Yoga, particularly its meditation paths, makes up the spiritual aspect of Ayurveda, while Ayurvedic diet, herb and lifestyle regimens make up the practical side of yogic spirituality. Yogic exercises to improve health are prescribed along with Ayurvedic health regimens for different constitutions. Yoga as a therapy for treating disease, whether physical or mental, is part of Ayurveda and is traditionally employed according to Ayurvedic diagnosis and recommendations. For those who want to benefit from Yoga and Ayurveda in the best possible manner, particularly as healing modalities, they should combine the two together in their daily lives. In this chapter, we will show how Yoga relates to Ayurveda and how yogic practices can be used as part of Ayurvedic healing.

Yoga and Ayurveda originated together as part of the

greater system of Vedic science passed on from the ancient seers, the rishis of the Himalayas. Both evolved from the same philosophy, culture and country. They both look at the human being from the same holistic angle and according to the same energetic language. Both are special ancient Vedic disciplines connected with related Vedic arts and sciences like music, dance, architecture and astrology. They can be easily integrated with one another.

Ayurveda is the science of life, helping us to realize our full human potential. According to Ayurveda, the human being consists of body, senses, mind and spirit. Ayurveda considers life a psychospiritual as well as a physical phenomenon. It aims at ending suffering so that every individual can actualize all four goals of life: Purpose, wealth, enjoyment and liberation (Dharma, Artha, Kama and Moksha). In dealing with liberation, Ayurveda moves into the field of Yoga and spirituality.

Yoga is the science of liberation, which comes through linking the individual self with the universal Self. Yoga expands the narrow, constricted, egoistic personality into the all-pervasive, eternal and blissful state of Pure Consciousness. While the aim of Yoga is to achieve liberation, it does not neglect the importance of health in the process. Without proper physical and mental health, we cannot effectively pursue the spiritual life or the material life. In moving into the field of health, Yoga enters the domain of Ayurveda.

Purity of body, mind and speech are essential for both physical health and spiritual liberation. Three important Sanskrit texts exist on the proper use of body, mind and speech, all attributed to the famous Yogi, Patanjali, who was not only the main teacher of the Yoga system, but a doctor and grammarian as well.

- *Yoga Sutras* of Patanjali - The classical work on the science of Yoga for purification of mind and realization of the Self.
- *Mahabhashya* of Patanjali - For purification of speech, an important work on Sanskrit language and grammar, the main commentary on Panini's grammar.

• *Charaka Samhita* of Charaka - For purification of the physical body, the main text of Ayurveda, with the commentary of Patanjali.

COMMON BASIS OF YOGA AND AYURVEDA

Both Ayurveda and Yoga look at the anatomy, physiology and treatment of the human body in the same manner. Both accept the Samkhya system of philosophy and its twenty-four tattvas. If we examine classical Yogic and Ayurvedic texts, we find the same terminology and approach. Both Ayurveda and Yoga are based upon the three gunas of Sattva, Rajas and Tamas. Both emphasize developing Sattva or the quality of purity in body and mind. Both use the theory of the five great elements, Ayurveda more for understanding the physical body and Yoga more for understanding the subtle body and the chakras.

Yoga textbooks advise us to study anatomy according to Ayurvedic principles, because unless one knows anatomy adequately, yogic practices cannot be properly performed. On the other hand, Ayurvedic textbooks, while explaining anatomy, point out that this study is good for practitioners of Yoga as well as physicians. Classical Yoga employs the dosha-tissue theory of Ayurveda for understanding the workings of the body. Similarly, it employs Ayurveda's taste-energy concept for understanding foods and medicines. That the health of the body depends upon the equilibrium of doshas, tissues and waste-materials is explained in the *Hatha Yoga Pradipika*, the most important Hatha Yoga text. For explaining human anatomy, both sciences employ the same terminology of blood vessels (Shira), nerves (Dhamanya), and tissues (Dhatus).

Yoga textbooks use the Ayurvedic terminology of the doshas and the digestive fire, Agni, for explaining the effects of postures and Pranayama. For describing the therapeutic usage of postures, they follow the Ayurvedic nomenclature for diseases. It has been clearly stated that when limitations to

Ayurvedic treatment are observed, one should consult a Yoga teacher. Similarly, side effects of improperly done Yoga practices should be treated by Ayurvedic remedies.

Ayurveda uses the concept of Agni-Soma emphasized in Yogic and Vedic texts. These two principles dominate all activities in the universe and in the human being. In the body, the right side is Sun-Agni dominant, while the left side is Moon-Soma dominant. This principle has been used for advising on right or left nostril breathing for certain diseases.

Vata, the principal energy of movement in the body, has a close relationship with Agni, the power of digestion. Both sciences explain that control of Vata is essential for controlling the power of digestion and ensuring health. Both Yoga and Ayurveda emphasize the role of Prana and its five subtypes (prana, apana, vyana, samana and udana). Both sciences teach that control over the sense organs is essential for happiness. Ayurveda describes wrong use of the senses as one of the main causes of disease. Yoga describes it as one of the main causes of spiritual bondage.

Ayurveda accepts the yogic principle that health of the body depends upon health and balance of the mind. The mind is inherently unstable like mercury and can be easily agitated and disturbed. It must be kept calm and controlled by restraining emotions like anger, fear and greed or it will lead not only to psychological but also to physical problems through inciting us to various wrong actions. Regular practice of Pranayama or yogic breathing is helpful for controlling the mind and is used for this purpose in Ayurveda.

There is a correlation between mind and Vata, the biological air-humor. A healthy mind can control Vata, and control over Vata keeps the mind under control. Mind and Vata are mutually related and their interaction determines how each functions. For example, when Vata or nervous energy is disturbed, the mind is disturbed. When the mind is calm, then our nerves will be calm. This concept is prominent in both sciences.

Ayurveda holds that health practices and therapies should

be adopted in a step-by-step manner. Similarly, the *Hatha Yoga Pradipika* states that postures and Pranayama should be undertaken gradually. Both systems aim at gradual and natural deep internal changes, not at forced, superficial and symptomatic results. Both Yoga and Ayurveda work with Nature in order to bring about change, uncovering her deeper forces and higher potentials. They do not follow the aggressive and intrusive model of biochemical medicine but channel the benefic energies from the Cosmos.

For maintenance of health, Yoga recommends a diet and lifestyle following one's Ayurvedic constitution. For mental health, Ayurveda recommends the ethical regimens like nonviolence and truthfulness and the other Yamas and Niyamas of Yoga. To gain the maximum benefits of Rasayana or rejuvenation treatment in particular, a person must follow such ethical disciplines. While explaining different exercises, Sushruta gives importance to yoga postures as the best general exercise for all types of people.

Both Yoga and Ayurveda advocate the use of diet, herbs, exercise, mantra and meditation for physical and mental health. In this regard, Ayurveda emphasizes employing these measures for treating diseases, while Yoga uses them for purification of the mind. Ayurveda contains specific psychological and spiritual therapies, emphasizing mantra, meditation and increasing Sattva, the clear quality of the mind, for mental and emotional disorders. These methods are yogic in nature.

LIBERATION, THE GOAL OF YOGA AND AYURVEDA

The great Ayurvedic doctor Charaka explains the law of similarity between the universe and the human being: The universe is the macrocosm, of which man is the microcosm or replica. The realization that the entire universe and the individual are one and the same is called "Satya-buddhi", which literally means "true intelligence." To bring this into function is the real goal of human life.

True intelligence (Satya-buddhi) brings about the realization of ultimate reality by showing us the eternal truth behind the changing appearances of the outer world. It eliminates all sorrow by showing its basic illusory nature and leads to liberation, which is inherent in our true Self. Charaka has explained that ego (self-centeredness) is the cause of all miseries. The moment true intelligence emerges, the soul or Atman transcends the ego and all worldly sufferings come to an end.

Action (pravritti) initiated by Karma (the results of past actions) is the root cause of all sorrow and keeps us bound to the cycle of time. True intelligence transcends all karmas and affords freedom from action (nivritti) by showing us that the eternal is ever present once we give up desire. This freedom from action, or the state of inaction, is the highest achievement. Detachment from action and ultimate realization (Moksha) are the same. Thus Charaka, like a yogic sage, describes the highest yogic achievement, knowledge of ultimate Truth, and teaches us how to achieve it.

Yogic science explains that in order to achieve liberation, one has to move inward from the physical body through the subtle bodies to the inner Self or Pure Consciousness.

- One proceeds from the physical sheath (Annamaya Kosha), made of the gross elements, to the Pranic or breath sheath (Pranamaya Kosha), composed of the vital force and its manifestations (the five pranas).
- Then one moves to the mental sheath (Manomaya Kosha) and the field of sensory impressions.
- From there, one goes to the wisdom sheath (Vijñanamaya Kosha), where the understanding of Truth abides.
- Finally, one enters the bliss sheath (Anandamaya Kosha), which holds our deepest joy and love.
- From there, one can transcend these sheaths and ultimately achieve liberation or the state of Pure Consciousness (Purusha).

Ayurveda helps us harmonize the physical, vital and mental sheaths. Yoga works on the deeper sheaths as well and takes us to the Purusha.

DIFFERENT METHODS OF YOGA

Yoga is the science that unites the outer being with the inner being. It gives control of our latent powers, which includes various extrasensory faculties. Many methods are described to achieve this goal. In this chapter, we will briefly discuss these different paths of Yoga.

Patanjali's Ashtanga Yoga

Ashtanga or Eightfold Yoga is the classical system of Yoga and aspects of it are found in most Yoga systems. Its eight limbs cover all other yogic approaches and provide a complete system of ethical, emotional, intellectual and spiritual training.

1. YAMA	Ten ethical rules that every Yoga practitioner should follow: Non-violence, truthfulness, non-stealing, control of sexual energy, forgiveness, patience, compassion, straight-forwardness, cleanliness and moderation in diet.
2. NIYAMA	The ten practices of self-discipline: Contentment, faith, charity, good company, modesty, control of the mind, chanting of mantras, devotion to God, and observation of vows.
3. ASANA	Yoga postures. In all, eighty-four varieties have been described. It must always be remembered that postures are not acrobatic exercises. Yoga postures require slow contraction and slow relaxation, with concentration on the breath.
4. PRANAYAMA	Various breathing techniques for controlling and developing the life-force, or Prana, so that we have the energy to achieve higher states of consciousness.

6. DHARANA	Centering and focusing the mind for concentration. The concentrated mind gains the ability to meditate and perceive Truth.
7. DHYANA	Meditation with concentration. Meditation, or dwelling on the nature of things, allows us to understand all the mysteries of existence.
8. SAMADHI	Integration of the perceiver and the perceived through continuous concentrated meditation. In this way, we become one with all that we give our attention to, discovering the unitary reality of Pure Consciousness.

Hatha Yoga

Hatha Yoga is perhaps the most well-known yogic approach in the Western world. Of all the types of Yoga, it is the one most directly concerned with the physical body, though it has much that goes beyond it as well. Because of its more physical side which emphasizes Yoga postures, it is also the most closely connected with Ayurveda.

The term Hatha is composed of two syllables "Ha" meaning the Sun or solar principle and "Tha" meaning the Moon or lunar principle. Our body is divided into two principles. The right side is Sun-dominant while the left is Moon-dominant. Health is maintained only when there is equilibrium between both parts. With the help of Hatha Yoga, one can achieve this equilibrium. Hatha Yoga prescribes the first five principles described in Ashtanga Yoga from Yama to Pratyahara. In addition, it emphasizes six special purificatory procedures (Shat Kriyas) which are described below.

Hatha Yoga provides many benefits for health and spiritual growth. It results in slimness of body, lustre of the face, clearness of voice, brightness of the eyes, freedom from disease, control over sexual energy, good digestive power, and purification of the Nadis or nerves. The individual becomes more active, alert, vital and energetic. Dullness and distraction (Tamas and

Rajas) decrease and clarity (Sattva) increases. This eventually results in the development of higher consciousness.

The initial stages of Hatha Yoga reduce the amount of inertia and attachment to the physical body. To aid in this effort, the individual must follow the rules of diet and behavior prescribed by this science. A person who wishes to practice Hatha Yoga seriously should avoid over-eating, overexertion, too much talking, excess public contact, and changeability of mind. He should practice Yoga postures, Pranayama and yogic purification practices culminating in meditation, following the ethical rules of Yama and Niyama. Hatha Yoga, therefore, is not just physical exercise. It is a way of life and leads us through various physical, mental and ethical disciplines to the ultimate Truth of reality. It is said to lead us to Raja Yoga or the higher Yoga, the union of the self with the Self.

Karma Yoga

Karma Yoga means service (Seva) or selfless work, action done with an attitude of detachment toward the fruits of one's efforts. One does one's best, giving total dedication to the work, without allowing the mind to be distracted by concern for personal gain. All misery and pain in life comes from attachment. If one works in such a selfless manner, one gains freedom from all sorrow. This requires surrender to the will of God, not as an external being, but as the true Self within the heart. Ayurveda as a path of service involves Karma Yoga.

Bhakti Yoga

Bhakti means devotion or unqualified love of God. Bhakti Yoga teaches us how to worship and meditate upon the Divine with love and affection so that we can become one with Him (or Her), either as formless or through various forms and personalities. Bhakti practices include devotional worship, mantra, chanting, singing and devotional dancing. With this type of Yoga, we gain control over emotional instabilities and find peace and contentment. Bhakti Yoga often goes along with Karma Yoga. Devotion allows us to perform all work as a service to the Divine.

Jñana Yoga

Jñana means knowledge of our True Nature, the Self beyond the mind, not just ordinary information and ideas. This form of Yoga teaches the process of right reasoning and Self-inquiry leading to thought-free meditation. With it, one gains acuity of mind in order to realize the ultimate Truth. It consists of listening to the Truth, thinking about it, and profound meditation bringing about its realization. Through it, we transcend our limited mortal nature and become one with the infinite and eternal consciousness behind the universe.

Raja Yoga

Raja Yoga means the "royal path" and is a many-sided, or integral, Yoga aiming at control of the mind through various procedures including service, devotion and wisdom. By controlling the mind, one gains an easy access to higher states of consciousness. Raja Yoga consists mainly of the inner aspects of Patanjali's Ashtanga Yoga system which comprise concentration, meditation, and realization (Dharana, Dhyana and Samadhi). However, it is also another name for Ashtanga Yoga as a whole.

Kundalini Yoga and Tantra

Kundalini Yoga teaches control over the dormant power of Kundalini, the psychic energy of transformation. Kundalini dwells at the base of the spine where the three psychic nerves (Ida, Pingala and Sushumna) come together. These three are reflected in the right and left sympathetic nerve chains and the spinal cord.

Kundalini, once awakened, rises through the chakras from the base of the spine (Muladhara Chakra) to the crown chakra in the head (Sahasrara). Along the way, it unfolds various powers, inner faculties and mystical experiences, giving us the actual experience of cosmic principles (tattvas) leading to ultimate Self-realization.

Kundalini is emphasized in various Tantric practices, which include a number of yogic approaches like Mantra Yoga and Laya Yoga (the Yoga of the sound current). These methods can be used for spiritual purposes or for gaining occult powers. Tantra emphasizes an energetic unfoldment of our various faculties and capacities, showing us how to use the forces of nature in order to go beyond them. In it, the worship of the Divine Mother, who represents this hidden power of nature and Kundalini, is central.

YOGA POSTURES FOR DIFFERENT CONSTITUTIONS

The most practical aspect of Yoga relative to Ayurveda is different Yoga postures for different Ayurvedic constitutions. Ayurveda deals with exercise, and Yoga postures are the ultimate form of exercise that it recommends. Yet Yoga, like Ayurveda, requires a certain life-regimen in order to be performed properly.

Yoga Postures for Vata Constitution

Vata people are inherently restless and changeable like the wind. They have trouble sitting still and staying focused. They benefit greatly from the calming and grounding effect of Yoga postures. Simple sitting poses such as those described below are best for them, though all types of asanas can be good for them if done gently and consistently.

SUKHASANA OR EASY POSTURE: Sit on a mat with the legs stretched out in front. Then bend the right leg at the knee and place the right foot under the left thigh by using your hand if required. Now bend the left leg and place the left foot under your right leg. Keep the vertebral column or spine erect. Extend both arms so that the wrists rest on the knees with palms turned upwards.

SIDDHASANA: Sit on a mat with the legs stretched out in front. Then bend the right leg at the knee and place the heel of the foot under the perineum. Now bend the left leg and bring the left heel against the pubic bone. Place both hands as in Sukhasana.

PADMASANA OR LOTUS POSTURE: First sit on a mat with your legs stretched out in front. Then, with the help of your hands, bring the right foot to rest on the left thigh, close to the hip joint, with the sole of the foot turned upwards and the heel near the middle of the abdomen. Then bend the left leg and bring the left foot onto the right thigh by crossing it over the right leg. Keep the spine erect and close the eyes. Both hands should be kept as in Sukhasana.

Yoga Postures for Pitta Constitution

Pitta people are determined, if not driven in their behavior, and easily get overheated, which can make them angry or irritable. Yoga postures can cool them down so that they avoid rash or inappropriate actions. This also helps them direct their sharp intelligence toward understanding themselves.

BHUJANGASANA OR THE COBRA POSE: Lay face down on the mat. Keep both legs together, chin touching the ground and the soles of the feet facing up. Keep the arms bent near the body, with the palms touching the ground near the shoulders. Raise the head slowly first and then the upper portion of the body until the navel area is about to lift above the ground. During this phase, no pressure should be placed on the hands. After maintaining this position for some time, return to the lying-down position.

VIPARITAKARINI: Lay flat on your back with legs stretched out and both hands near the body. Keeping the knees stiff, slowly raise both legs to an angle of forty-five degrees over the torso. Keep the position for some time, then return to normal position.

SARVANGASANA OR SHOULDER STAND: Lay flat on your back with legs stretched out. Then first come to the position of Viparitakarini. Raise the legs further up to a ninety degree angle. Now raise the buttocks and the trunk as well, using the support of the arms and elbows, without lifting the head. Rest the elbows on the ground firmly and support the back with both palms. Straighten the trunk with the hands until the chin is well set in at the suprasternal notch. Maintain this position and then slowly return to normal.

HALASANA OR PLOUGH POSE: Raise your legs until they are ninety degrees, as in the shoulder stand. Then slowly swing them over your head until they are parallel to the floor or further, till the toes touch the ground. Keep the legs straight and the palms of your hands flat on the floor with the arms stretched for support. Maintain this position and then slowly return to normal position.

Yoga Postures for Kapha Constitution

Kapha people easily develop congestion or stagnation in the body, especially in the lungs. Yoga postures help open up their energy and remove these obstructions. This brings more movement to both body and mind so that they can change their lives in a positive direction. Along with asanas, Kapha types benefit from strong Pranayama to get their internal energies moving.

PASCHIMOTANASANA: Sit on the mat with your legs stretched out in front. Bend forward from the hip hinge, keeping the spine straight and rest the hands on the legs or ankles or hook your index fingers around the big toes. Slowly stretch further forward, extending the spine, so that the trunk is stretched along the thighs and the face rests on the knees. Maintain and then return to normal position.

VIRABHADRASANA: Stand straight. Spread your feet approximately five feet apart. Raise your arms out to the sides at shoulder level. Turn your right foot, knee and leg 90 degrees to the right. Turn your left foot in slightly by moving the left heel out. Stand with the weight on the outsides of your feet, arches lifting. Bend your right knee to 90 degrees, shin vertical to the floor with the hips facing forward. Keep your left leg and knee straight. Your lower back lengthens down as your chest opens forward and up. Stretch out through the arms and hands while keeping your shoulders down away from your ears. Then return to standing pose. Repeat to the other side.

THE SIX YOGIC PURIFICATION PRACTICES

Internal cleansing is necessary to remove physical toxins and negative emotions so that we can be happy and healthy. For purification of body and mind, both Yoga and Ayurveda have several special methods. Ayurveda emphasizes Pancha Karma, the five purification practices of emesis, purgation, enemas, nasya and blood purification, as already discussed. Yoga has its purification methods as well, which can be used along with these.

Hatha Yoga Pradipika explains that Ayurvedic oil and sweating therapies (snehana and swedana) should be done prior to Yogic purification practices and that Ayurvedic enemas and nasal medications (Basti and Nasya) should be done every day by advanced Hatha Yogis. It describes the six yogic purificatory actions (Shuddhi Kriyas), useful for purifying the body:

| 1. Kapalabhati | 2. Neti | 3. Dhouti | 4. Nauli | 5. Trataka | 6. Basti |

In the section on Pranayama, we will discuss the technique of Kapalabhati. In this chapter we will discuss the remaining practices.

NETI – NASAL CLEANSING

Neti consists of various methods for cleansing the nose and nasal passages. These open the region of the head and sinuses and the higher chakras, improving the flow of Prana. Four types of Neti exist:

1. Jala Neti – Water cleansing
2. Sutra Neti – Cleansing with a cloth
3. Dugha Neti – Cleansing with milk
4. Ghrita Neti – Cleansing with ghee or clarified butter

Jala Neti is the most important and commonly used of these four. It requires a special vessel called a "Neti pot" which is used to pour water through the nose. It can be purchased at Ayurvedic stores or wherever yogic implements are sold.

Water Cleansing or Jala Neti

Fill a Neti pot with lukewarm water and add about an eighth of a teaspoon of salt. Hold the pot in your right hand. Insert the nozzle of the pot into the right nostril. Keep the mouth open to allow free breathing through it. Tilt your head first slightly backwards, then forward and sideways to the left so that the water from the pot enters the right nostril and comes out through the left by the force of gravity. Let the water flow till the pot is empty. Should any congestion in the head prevent the flow of water, hold the position for a short while and the passage may open, or tilt the head down and let the water flow out the same nostril and try again.

Repeat the same process on the left side. When the process is complete, remove any remaining water in the nasal passages with gentle forced exhalations through the nostrils. It is better to exhale through both nostrils because this helps regulate the pressure in the head. In this cleansing process, mucus and other impurities will be discharged.

By slightly bending the head back, the water will flow down into the mouth, where you can spit it out. This is called "Usah Pana", which is very beneficial and can be practiced every morning before sunrise.

Feel free to adjust the amount of salt according to what is comfortable for you. Too much salt may cause a burning sensation in the nose, too little can irritate the mucous membranes. The temperature of the water can also be adjusted; usually slightly warm is good, not hot nor cold.

Spring or distilled water should be used as tap water, which is chlorinated, can be irritating. Herbal decoctions can be used instead of water for specific therapeutic purposes, but should contain some salt as well.

Sutra Neti or Rubber Catheter Neti

This procedure is a little more complex and technical and should be learned from one who knows it. Insert the blunt end of a thin soft rubber catheter from the front horizontally into the right nostril. The catheter should be previously lubricated with sesame or another oil.

Push it along the floor of the nose until the tip is felt in the back of the throat. Insert the right index and the middle fingers through the mouth and catch the tip of the catheter at the back of the throat. Pull it out through the mouth and gently massage the nasal passage by catching the two ends of the tube. Remove the catheter through the nose. Repeat the same procedure on the left side after lubricating the catheter again.

This process requires some skill and should not be done unless one is proficient at Jala Neti. It may cause nausea or vomiting in some people and should be done with care.

Dugha Neti and Ghrita Neti

The procedure for these is the same as for Jala Neti, only instead of water, milk (dugha) and ghee (ghrita) are used. Medicated ghees, medicated oils and herbal decoctions in milk can also be used in this manner.

DHOUTI — CLEANSING THE STOMACH

This is a technical yogic procedure that cleanses the intestinal tract down to the stomach. There are three types of Dhouti:

- Jala or Vamana Dhouti - Water cleansing
- Vastra Dhouti - Cleansing with a cloth
- Danda Dhouti - Cleansing with a tube

While we mention the procedure for performing types of Dhouti that require swallowing a cloth or rubber tube, we do not recommend trying them on your own. They should be done only after careful and experienced instruction from a competent Yoga teacher. Some people have harmed themselves by attempting these practices without the proper guidance.

Jala Dhouti or Vamana Dhouti - Water Cleansing

This is simply vomiting with the help of salt water. Sit on your heels and drink lukewarm salt water until you can take no more or until there is a sensation of vomiting. Churn your stomach with twisting exercises.

Stand with feet together and bend forward, forming an angle of about ninety degrees, and vomit. If you cannot vomit easily, tickle the back of your throat with your finger until the sensation of vomiting occurs causing all the water to be vomited out.

This method is essentially the same practice as Vamana or emetic therapy in Ayurveda. Similar herbal substances can be used to increase its therapeutic effectiveness. It can be a helpful daily practice done early in the morning to remove excess Kapha.

Vastra Dhouti - Cleansing with a Cloth

This method uses a cloth for cleansing the stomach. Take a very soft cloth four inches wide and seven feet long. Put it into water or milk so that it becomes very soft. Then slowly swallow it until one end reaches the stomach and the other end is still in the mouth. After a short time, slowly bring out the cloth while exhaling, without using any force. This procedure is called Vastra Dhouti. During swallowing or while taking out the cloth, if it sticks, drink some water and this will help release the muscle spasm.

Swallowing the cloth may cause some nausea or vomiting reflexes. It should not be done by those with sensitive or nervous stomachs, like Vata types, nor should it be attempted by those who have not first mastered the Jala Dhouti or water cleansing. Be sure to use a cloth made of natural fibers like cotton that does not contain any harmful dyes.

Danda Dhouti

Here a rubber tube is used to clean the stomach. Drink lukewarm salt water as in Jala Dhouti. Then take a flexible rubber tube about half an inch in diameter and about three feet long.

Slowly start to swallow the tube. When it reaches the stomach, bend forward. All of the swallowed water will come out by a siphoning action.

This method is yet more difficult and should not be done by those who are not proficient in the other two forms of Dhouti. Please do not attempt it without due instruction and caution.

NAULI

Nauli is an abdominal action that requires isolation and rolling manipulation of the abdominal muscles. It requires personal instruction in order to be performed properly. Several types are listed below.

UDDIYANA BANDHA – Stand with a slight forward bend of the trunk with palms on the thighs and the feet about three feet apart.

Exhale completely by vigorously contracting the muscles of the abdomen. At this time the chest should also contract. Then press the hands against the thighs and at the same time try to tighten the muscles of the neck and shoulder. Carry out a vigorous mock-inhalation by raising the ribs without actually allowing the air to flow into the lungs. Relax the muscles of the abdomen. Automatically the diaphragm will rise up, producing a concave depression of the abdomen. This result is called Uddiyana.

In this condition, when the breath is entirely exhaled, quickly push out and pull in the abdominal muscles alternately. Continue as long as you can hold your breath. Count the number of contractions. This process is called "Agnisara Kriya." It is very useful for increasing the digestive power.

MADHYAMA NAULI – Maintaining Uddiyana, give a forward and downward push to the abdominal point just above the pelvic bone in the mid-line, where the two rectus abdominous muscles originate. This push brings about the concentration of these muscles, which stand out in the center, leaving the other muscles of the abdominal wall in a relaxed condition. This is Madhyama Nauli.

DAKSHINA AND VAMA NAULI – Dakshina means right. For right side Nauli, one has to contract the right rectus abdominous muscle, leaving the other muscles, including the left rectus abdominous, relaxed.

Vama means left. For left side Nauli, the opposite procedure should be done, contracting the left rectus abdominous muscle and leaving the right relaxed.

NAULI CHALANA – After gaining full control over the first three types, one should roll the rectus abdominous muscles clockwise and counter-clockwise. This rolling is called Nauli Chalana.

TRATAKA – CLEANSING THE EYES

Our eyes easily become strained, congested or simply sensitive. Yoga provides special exercises that tone the eyes, improve vision, aid in concentration and help open our inner sight as well. Trataka is a procedure for cleansing the eyes that can be done simply, safely and effectively on a regular basis by everyone. Sit in any meditative posture comfortably with an erect spine.

Arrange a burning candle or ghee lamp with the flame set at the same height as the eyes and at a distance of about three feet. Gaze at the flame without blinking your eyes. Try to hold your concentration and ignore any irritation and watering of the eyes. With practice, your gaze will become steady, calming your mind as well. Try to relax the eyes in this focused position. Increase your practice slowly, starting with thirty seconds and increasing the duration by ten seconds per week.

Trataka improves our visual capacity and can be helpful in treating headaches and nervous problems. A ghee flame gives better results than a candle. For this, take a ghee lamp or any small metal bowl. Fill it with ghee and add a wick made of cotton. To make a cotton wick, take any ball of cotton and stretch and roll it into the size and shape of a wick.

Pranayama

"Prana" means breath and "Ayama" means pause or retention. Hence, Pranayama literally means retention of breath. However, Pranayama should not be equated simply with merely holding one's breath or failing to breathe, which is debilitating. Pranayama means creating a balance of energies through which our vitality is extended and our breath is deepened. Through Pranayama, one slows down and extends the breath so that one's inner Prana or higher life-force can manifest. This also aids in slowing down and calming the mind. The practice of Pranayama balances Prana and Apana and normalizes Vata. In this way, it is useful in treating many diseases. The use of Prana for healing, or Pranic healing, is an important aspect of Ayurveda.

While there are many types of Pranayama, they are usually classified in four groups based upon the nature of the retention:

- Retention after expiration (rechaka), called outer retention (bahya kumbhaka)
- Retention after inspiration (puraka), called inner retention (abhyantara kumbhaka)
- Retention made at once
- Retention after many inhalations and exhalations

These last two forms of retention are called "kevala kumbhaka". Thus, the action of Pranayama consists of four phases:

- Inspiration – Puraka
- Inner retention – Abhyantara Kumbhaka
- Expiration – Rechaka
- Outer retention – Bahya Kumbhaka

Proportion
The proportion of inhalation, exhalation and retention is important in determining the strength and nature of Pranayama. A beginner should practice Pranayama with a one-to-two ratio of inhalation and exhalation; that is, with exhalation held twice

as long as inhalation. After proficiency in this is gained, one should practice with a proportion of inhalation one, internal retention two, exhalation two, and external retention two.

The ideal proportion is inhalation one, internal retention four, exhalation two, and external retention four, but this takes some time to be able to do with ease and requires the development of much internal strength. In Pranayama there should be no straining to achieve results but a natural deepening of the breath by letting go of strain and tension.

Technique

Pranayama is best learned by direct instruction from a qualified teacher. The following guidelines should not substitute for that. To practice Pranayama, sit in Padmasana (lotus posture), Siddhasana, Svastikasana, or any other comfortable seated pose. The place of practice should be well ventilated but the draft of air should not come directly toward the body. Open air and a calm and quiet place are preferable.

Certain types of Pranayama require closing alternate nostrils. For this, the right palm is first spread out. The index and middle fingers are turned down, lightly resting just above the bridge of the nose. The thumb is placed on the bridge of the nose at the right nostril and the pinky and ring fingers together on the left. Then alternately, the thumb or other two fingers are used to close and open the right or left nostrils for Pranayama.

Types of Pranayama

Hatha Yoga Pradipika has described eight different types of Pranayama, which we will briefly discuss, with Kapalabhati making nine.

1. Ujjayi	2. Kapalabhati	3. Bhastrika
4. Suryabhedana	5. Sitkari	6. Shitali
7. Bhramari	8. Murccha	9. Plavini

1. Ujjayi

The meaning of this word is "to pronounce loudly" or "what leads to success and victory." In this type of Pranayama, the breath is drawn in through both the nostrils. During inhalation, the glottis is to be partially closed, which will produce sound. Retention should then be done with Jalandhara bandha (chin lock) and then both nostrils should be closed. Then exhalation should be done through the left nostril. The proportion between inhalation and exhalation should be one to two and retention should be done until there is no sensation of suffocation.

2. Kapalabhati

This is also one of the procedures for cleansing the nasal passages in the head. The actual meaning is "what makes the head shine." Strictly speaking, it is not a type of Pranayama because it does not involve retention of the breath.

First, a forceful exhalation should be done which is a little deeper than ordinary breathing. At this time, the front abdominal muscles are suddenly and vigorously contracted. Then inhalation should be performed by simply relaxing the abdominal muscles. In this procedure, retention is not to be done. The beginner should start with eleven expulsions in each round. With each expiration, a stroke is delivered to the center of the abdomen, which helps to spiritually activate the nervous system.

3. Bhastrika

Bhastrika is characterized by a quick expulsion of the breath producing a sound like a bellow. It differs little from Kapalabhati. There are four varieties of Bhastrika. The first type starts out with several quick rounds of Kapalabhati. After the last expulsion of Kapalabhati, a very deep inhalation is done followed by internal retention. Then exhalation should be done slowly, followed by external retention. This entire procedure completes one round of Bhastrika.

The only difference between the first and second type is that the inhalation-internal retention, exhalation-external retention procedure for the second type should be done only with the right nostril. In the third variety, quick respirations are done through the right nostril, keeping the left closed. After some rounds, the inhalation should be done through the same nostril. Then retention is done and exhalation through the left nostril.

In the fourth variety, quick inhalation through the right nostril and quick retention through the left nostril should be done until one is fatigued. Then the deepest possible inspiration through the right nostril should be done and, after retention, exhalation should be done through the left nostril.

4. Suryabhedana

In this type of Pranayama, one breathes in through the Sun-dominant right nostril, then retention should be done until there is perspiration, followed by exhalation through the Moon-dominant left nostril. This increases heat in the body. The opposite type of Pranayama, Chandrabhedana, or breathing in through the left nostril and out through the right, increases coolness.

5. Sitkari

Sit in a comfortable posture with an erect spine. First do exhalation from both nostrils. Fold the tongue backwards and press the tip of the tongue to the roof of the mouth, leaving a small opening on either side of the tongue. Carry out inhalation through these side openings. During this time, a hissing sound like "sit" is made. After completing inhalation, the tongue should be withdrawn, the mouth closed, and then retention should be performed followed by exhalation.

6. Shitali

This type of Pranayama produces a cooling effect in the body. Hence, it is called Shitali, which means "cooling." For practicing this, fold up the sides of a partially protruding tongue so as to form a long narrow tube resembling the beak of a bird. Further narrow this passage by pressing your lips around the tongue. Take an inhalation and perceive the cooling effect of the air as it passes through the tongue. Then close the mouth and do retention. Exhalation should be done through both nostrils.

7. Bhramari

In this type of Pranayama, a quick forced inspiration is used to produce a humming sound like a bee. Hence, it is called as Bhramari, which means "the buzzing of a bee." While doing inhalation, lift the soft palate and draw it toward the nasal part of the pharynx. This produces a sound due to the vibration of the soft palate. Then retention of the breath should be done as usual. Exhalation requires the same movement of the soft palate.

8. Murccha

Murccha means "temporary loss of consciousness." First inhalation should be done. At the end of inhalation, Jalandhara bandha or the chin lock should be done, followed by retention. This position should be maintained just long enough so that it produces a sensation leading to loss of awareness. Then the breath should be exhaled completely.

9. Plavini

With this type of Pranayama, one can easily "float on the water" for a long time, which is the meaning of Plavini. First, the person should try to swallow air into the stomach. After filling the stomach with plenty of air, he should take a very deep inhalation followed by retention. After retaining the breath as much as possible, exhalation should be done slowly.

Results of Pranayama

Pranayama involves conscious rhythmic breathing with retention. Normally we breathe in and breathe out every three or four seconds. With Pranayama, the breathing cycle extends to over a minute. Thus, respiratory exertion is reduced, which benefits vitality and helps increase the span of life. It is observed that athletes who do heavy exercise with short and quick breathing have comparatively short life spans, irrespective of a beautifully built body and admirable features. This is the case with boxers, weight lifters and wrestlers, who spend much time in excited states of mind with quick and short breathing. On the other hand, yogis can live long because their breath is long and deep.

According to Ayurveda, Pranayama is not only the exercise of the lungs but also an exercise for all the hollow organs in the body. The lung tissue taxes the circulation when it is in an active stage during normal respiration. With Pranayama, it is rendered almost at rest by sustained relaxation. At the same time, the rhythmic contraction and relaxation of the major hollow organs in the abdominal area allows them to discard waste-material that has accumulated. Thus, Pranayama has an indirect cleansing effect on the hollow organs of the body. It helps the propulsion of doshas toward the digestive tract for their elimination.

Due to the rhythm created by Pranayama, the lungs and other major hollow organs engaged in the process can drive out their waste products and keep themselves clean. If we compare this with the low and high tides of the sea, then we will understand why the sea can throw off any material put into it. Lakes, on the other hand, do not have such rhythm, hence everything put in goes to the bottom and remains there as silt.

Whenever the digestive tract or any hollow organ is filled with excessive fluid, as when we have overeaten, when the bladder is full, or when there is excessive fluid in the blood stream, as in congestive cardiac failure, there is always dyspnea or difficulty in breathing. The health-promoting effects of Pranayama are not restricted to the lungs. If the lungs are kept clean by a process of conscious and rhythmic breathing, other hollow organs can be kept healthy, and through them the entire body can be cleansed.

ALTERNATE NOSTRIL BREATHING IN AYURVEDIC TREATMENT

Alternate nostril breathing (Suryabhedana and Chandrabhedana) is the most important Pranayama technique used in Ayurveda. To understand the reason for this, let us consider anatomy according to Yoga. The Pingala Nadi, or right subtle nerve channel, starts from the right side of the perineum and crosses the vertebral column from left to right at each chakra, ultimately ending in the right nostril. The Ida, or left subtle nerve channel, starts from the left side and, crossing the vertebral column twice, ends in the left nostril.

The right side of the trunk contains the main organs responsible for digestion - the liver and pancreas. On the other hand, the organs responsible for nourishment - the heart and the stomach - are located on the left side of the trunk. Some Yoga texts place a secondary solar chakra on the right side near the liver and a secondary lunar chakra on the left side near the stomach.

Our breath predominates in one nostril at a time, alternating from one to the other at different times during the day. Right-nostril breathing, which has a heating effect, is observed more when the environment or body conditions are cool. When the body and outside conditions are comparatively hot, breathing is mainly from the left nostril, which has a cooling effect. Because the right side of the body is predominantly hot, right-nostril breathing compensates for cold. Similarly, because the left side of the body is predominantly cool, left-nostril breathing compensates for heat. The right side of the body, predominant in the solar or heat principle, is catabolic (stimulating and reducing) in nature, while the left side, predominant in the lunar or cold principle, is anabolic (building or sedating).

Therefore, if only left-nostril breathing is continued for a long time, it has a cooling effect on the body, while right-nostril breathing alone is heating. Hence, patients suffering from cold diseases like obesity, edema and muscle stiffness should emphasize right nostril breathing. In these patients, close the left nostril with the help of a cotton swab. Initially, this practice should be done for thirty seconds only. It should be increased slowly to two or three minutes at a time, and then longer.

On the other hand, patients suffering from hot or catabolic diseases like fevers, wasting diseases or paralysis along with loss of body weight, should emphasize left nostril breathing. Left-nostril breathing is also useful in conditions of hyperactivity of the mind including insomnia, restlessness and nervous agitation. Right-nostril breathing is useful in hypoactive conditions of the mind including sleepiness, dullness and fatigue.

YOGA PROCEDURES ACCORDING TO CONSTITUTION

Yoga procedures should be done according to constitution and should be included as part of our daily and seasonal lifestyle regimens. If we practice Yoga without knowing our constitution, the results will be lessened and can even be harmful.

Generally, yoga practices, which generally aim at creating lightness in the body and space in the mind, tend to increase Vata that is itself composed of air and ether elements. However, yoga practices that are heating can increase Pitta. Yoga in general decreases Kapha, particularly pranayama.

Yoga Procedures for Vata

Vata people require calming and warming Yoga practices so as not to exhaust them. They should perform sitting postures like Svastikasana, Padmasana, or Sukhasana postures every day for increasing stability. Also useful are Vajrasana and Siddhasana. Postures that afford the major muscle tissue areas a calm and restricted action are best. To control Vata, the practitioner should meditate in these postures as well. Meditation done properly controls the mind, which in turn controls Vata.

For Pranayama, Vatas should practice mainly right-nostril breathing, inhaling with the right nostril and exhaling with the left every day for ten to fifteen minutes. This compensates for coldness due to Vata and is very beneficial. They should not carry out stronger purification procedures like Dhouti, but Jala Neti and Trataka are good. For them, oil enema treatment

(Basti) is best because it alleviates constipation, their most common complaint.

Deep relaxation is a key to reducing high Vata, so all yoga postures should end with relaxing poses like Savasana (corpse pose) to make sure that no Vata has accumulated during the practice.

Yoga Procedures for Pitta

Pitta people have excess hot and warm qualities in their body. To compensate for this, they should follow Yoga procedures that create coolness. Shitali inhalation and Sitkari exhalation have this effect, as does lunar or left nostril breathing.

According to the yogic understanding of the body, the Sun principle in the body is located around the umbilicus, while that of the Moon is around the soft palate in the mouth, where salivary secretions constantly take place. It is thought that the Sun, with its upward moving heat, works to reduce the activity of the Moon in the soft palate. Putting the body regularly in the simple inverted pose (Viparitakarini), the shoulder stand (Sarvangasana), or plough pose (Halasana) helps protect the lunar principle from the harmful effects of the solar principle and creates coolness in the body. In these postures, the positions of the Sun and the Moon are reversed. This is naturally beneficial for Pitta types.

Pitta people also benefit from postures that slowly massage the liver and spleen area, which is the main site of Pitta in the body. For this purpose, they should do the bow pose (Dhanurasana), cobra pose (Bhujagasana) and fish pose (Matsyasana). These postures help eliminate excess Pitta from the digestive system.

Yoga Procedures for Kapha

Kapha people usually have slow digestion and a low metabolism. To stimulate their digestive capacity, procedures having an action on the navel region (where Agni is situated) are very useful. These are Nauli, Agnisara, or Nauli chalana. Purificatory procedures like Neti and Dhouti are especially helpful for them, but as always, should be done with caution.

Paschimottanasana is the most beneficial of the Yoga postures, as is Yogamudra. General yogic stretching, particularly
of the chest and arms, is also very helpful for Kaphas (such
as occurs in the Virabhadrasana posture). Paschimottanasana
relieves Kapha from its place of accumulation in the upper
body. More active asanas are good for Kapha types for promoting circulation and preventing Kapha type stagnation from
developing in the body.

The Ujjayi type of Pranayama, if done regularly, as well
as solar or right nostril breathing, reduces excess Kapha in
the body by creating heat. Bhastrika and other fiery type
Pranayama can strongly reduce Kapha but should be done with
care. Generally, Kapha types need to emphasize Pranayama
and make sure to breathe deeply during calmer yoga postures
to keep their energy moving internally.

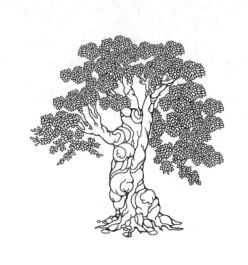

Dual Dosha Diet

By Dr. Marc Halpern

While some individuals have a constitution dominant in one doshic type, most individuals have a significant blending of the three doshas making up their constitutions. It is this blending which makes each of us different and each person's path toward optimal health unique.

When we are healthy, each person's diet should be in harmony with their constitution and adjusted slightly for seasonal considerations. When we are unhealthy, our diets should be according to the nature of our imbalance. Most commonly, we move out of balance in a similar pattern as our constitution, however, this is not always true. Thus, careful assessment is needed to separate ones constitution (prakruti) from one's imbalance (vikruti).

The practice of Ayurveda is an attempt to understand as specifically as possible the nature of a person, the nature of the imbalances present and the nature of the remedies most applicable to them. The greater the depth of specificity and understanding, the more individualized a program can be and the greater the likelihood that a person will thrive on their program.

Designing food programs according to one dosha gives us only three food programs to choose from. Adding dual and tridoshic diets increases our dietary choices to seven. It should be understood that a person's diet could be further tailored to be more specific once the exact balance of the doshas which are at play has been determined. That type of specificity usually requires an evaluation by a trained practitioner.

Dual doshic diets emphasize foods that are best for both constitutions and recommend only modest intake of foods that are good for one type but harmful for another. Foods that are harmful to both types should be avoided. Tridoshic diets emphasize foods that balance all three doshas and avoid foods which imbalance all three.

Vata-Pitta

Vata is composed of air and ether and has the qualities of being light, dry and cold. Pitta is composed primarily of fire and contains a little bit of water, which gives it an oily quality. In bringing balance to both doshas at one time, we look at which qualities and elements the doshas have in common and which are different. Vata and Pitta share the quality of lightness. They are not composed of similar elements, but rather have in common the absence of earth in their make up. Thus, we see that a diet which is heavier or nourishing and which contains earth will bring the greatest balance to both doshas.

Individuals with a Vata - Pitta imbalance often appear light (characteristic of both doshas) and warm (characteristic of Pitta). Their skin tends to be dry (characteristic of Vata). Their diet must be heavy to balance the lightness, cool to balance the build up of heat, and moist or oily to balance the dryness.

Sweet taste is composed of earth and water. It is the heaviest, most nourishing of all tastes. The earth component in sweet taste brings stability to both Vata and Pitta, while its watery quality brings moistness to Vata and is somewhat neutral to Pitta. It is a cooling taste making it even more ideal for this dual combination. The sweet taste may best be found in grains, dairy, meats and nuts. Emphasizing these foods is most important. Intense sweeteners such as sugar should not be used in abundance as they agitate all three doshas when taken in excess.

Foods that emphasize the bitter and pungent tastes are the lightest. The bitter taste is composed of air and ether while the pungent taste is composed of fire and ether. As neither has much substance, they should not constitute a major portion of the diet. Leafy greens and hot spices are good examples of such foods.

Tastes best for this constitution in order from best to worst: Sweet, astringent, sour, salty, bitter and pungent.

Vata-Kapha

These two doshas at first appear diametrically opposed to one another. Careful examination reveals that some commonalties can be found and this is the basis of designing a proper food program. Kapha is made up of earth and water. It is heavy, moist and cold. Vata is made up of air and ether. It is light, dry and cold. In addition to having in common a cold nature, they also share a lack of fire in their compositions. Thus, a dual dosha diet emphasizes balancing their cold nature by adding fire.

Individuals with Vata-Kapha imbalances often appear heavy (a Kapha quality) and experience anxiety (a Vata characteristic). Their skin tends to be dry, but may be moist, and it feels cool to the touch. The diet must be light enough to slowly reduce Kapha but nourishing enough to satisfy Vata. Above all, the diet should consist of warm foods.

Adding warm spices to a diet is the surest way of introducing fire to a meal. Cooking the food also imparts fire and makes food more digestible. Thus, the Vata-Kapha food program emphasizes cooked foods that are spiced moderate to hot.

Tastes that contain fire will be the best for those trying to balance Vata and Kapha. The pungent taste, which contains fire and air is the best. The fire element is best for both Vata and Kapha; the air component in excess can aggravate Vata. Therefore, while pungent taste is the best food, food should not be taken extremely hot. Rather, it should be spiced from moderate to hot. Fire can also be found in the sour and salty tastes. Only moderate use of these tastes is recommended as they contain other elements that may cause imbalances.

Nourishment is needed to satisfy Vata. A lack of nourishment, either physical or emotional, creates greater anxiety and may provoke excessive eating. Thus, small to moderate amounts of heavier foods are needed. While the sweet taste (earth and water) is the heaviest and most nourishing, the sour taste (fire and earth) is also nourishing and has the benefit of containing fire. Hence, moderate use of the sour taste is beneficial.

As both constitutions are aggravated by the cold quality, cold foods should be used only in the smallest amounts. Bitter taste is made up of air and ether. While it brings balance to Kapha, it is very disturbing to Vata. As Vata disturbances are most often at the root of Vata-Kapha imbalances, this taste should be used the least.

> Tastes best for this constitution in order from best to worst: Pungent, sour, salty, astringent, sweet and bitter.

Pitta-Kapha

Pitta is composed primarily of fire and some water. It is hot, light and a little moist or slightly oily. Kapha is composed of water and earth. It is cold, heavy and moist or damp. What they have in common is the element water and the moist quality it creates. This is what becomes disturbed when both doshas combine in a state of imbalance. Looking closer at the two doshas, we also see that they have in common a lack of ether and air. Thus, a dual doshic diet for these individuals will emphasize dry foods rich in these elements.

People of Pitta-Kapha imbalance appear heavy (a Kapha quality), hot (a Pitta quality) and moist or oily (common to both). Hence, their food program is designed to be light, cool and dry in order to bring balance to both doshas. Hence, light foods such as salads and vegetables taken uncooked are ideal and should make up a large portion of the diet.

Bitter taste is the best taste for a person trying to balance Pitta and Kapha. Composed of air and ether, it is dry, light and cool and thus, it is the perfect complement. Bitter foods include many leafy green vegetables. The astringent taste is the next best. Consisting of air and earth, the dry quality of air balances out the moist/oily imbalance while also providing a light quality to counteract the heaviness of the earth element. Hence, it is dry and not too heavy or light. Fire, the hottest element should be limited. It is contained within the salty, sour and pungent tastes. Foods should only be spiced mild to moderately hot. The water element, having the qualities of heaviness and moistness, should be used most sparingly. It is contained within the sweet and salty tastes.

Tastes best for this constitution in order from best to worst: Bitter, astringent, pungent, sweet, sour and salty.

The Sannipatika and Tridoshic diet

Trying to reduce all three doshas is quite a balancing act. There is no one taste, element or quality that balances all three doshas. However, some foods, because of their unique balance of the elements and tastes, have a neutral effect on each of the doshas. These foods are understood to be tridoshic. Therefore, they are not strong agents for correcting imbalances and they do not cause aggravation. These foods are ideal for a healthy person with a tridoshic constitution.

Individuals with a tridoshic constitution usually share characteristics of all three types equally. Most commonly, they exhibit the qualities of heaviness (a Kapha quality), warmth (a

Pitta quality) and dryness (a Vata quality). For example, their bones are dense, their complexion is ruddy and the skin and membranes are dry. Hence, their ideal food program will usually emphasize light, cool and moist qualities. Those individuals with a tridoshic constitution most often need to consume a wide variety of foods emphasizing all six tastes in reasonably equal proportions in order to maintain balance.

For tridoshic individuals who are in reasonably good balance, the influence of the seasons becomes very important. During the winter and early spring (Kapha season), the diet should be lighter, warmer and drier. During the late spring and summer (Pitta season), the diet should be cooler. During the fall and early winter (Vata season), the diet should be heavier, warmer and more oily.

Some individuals develop imbalances in all three doshas. This is called sannipatika. In these individuals, qualities from all three doshas are out of balance. There are many possible presentations of qualities and thus the diet must be specifically tailored. Healing from these imbalances is more difficult and requires the care of a skilled clinical practitioner.

Dietary Progams for Dual Doshas

Listed below are recommended dietary programs for each of the dual doshas.

Foods listed as "best" can be eaten without reservation on a daily basis. Individuals who are sick should consume only those foods on this list. These foods are the most ideal as they are either close to, or perfectly balanced for both doshas.

Foods listed as "small amounts" can be eaten in small portions fairly often or in larger portions once or twice each week. Eating a wide variety of these foods is better than an abundance of just one. Over-reliance upon these foods can cause an imbalance.

Foods listed as "avoid" should be eaten only on rare occasions and can be eaten once each month. They either cause an imbalance in both doshas or very significantly disturb one of the doshas.

1. Vata-Pitta Food Program

BASIC PRINCIPLES

Qualities to reduce: Hot, light and dry
Best Taste: Sweet
Small Amounts: Astringent, sour
Worst Tastes: Salty, pungent and bitter

FOOD GROUPS

Grains: It is best to eat these as cooked grains or un-yeasted breads.

Best	Wheat, cooked oats, white basmati rice
Small Amounts	Amaranth, barley, rice (brown or white, short or long grain), millet, quinoa, rye
Avoid	Buckwheat, corn flour products, dry oats

Dairy: It is best to use raw or organic milk. Milk should be taken warm with a small amount of spices such as ginger and cardamom.

Best	Butter, cottage cheese, cream cheese, ghee, milk (whole), paneer (farmer's) cheese
Small Amounts	Buttermilk, hard unsalted cheeses, kefir, sour cream, yogurt
Avoid	Ice cream, frozen yogurt

Sweeteners: Overuse of any sweetener
will eventually cause an imbalance.

Best	Honey (fresh), maltose, maple syrup, maple sugar, rice syrup
Small Amounts	Date sugar, dextrose, fructose, grape sugar, molasses, sucanat (jaggery)
Avoid	White table sugar

Oils: Oils are very important and should be used
abundantly if the skin is dry. They alleviate dryness
and are generally heavy and nourishing.

Best	Avocado, coconut, ghee, olive oil, sunflower
Small Amounts	Sesame, almond, castor, flaxseed, corn, soy
Avoid	Safflower, margarine, mustard, peanut, lard, canola

Fruit: Fruit is best when it is well ripened and sweet.
This will bring balance to both doshas. In general, due to its
lightness, fruit should be consumed in moderation.

Best	Apricots, avocado, bananas (sweet), black berries, blueberries, cantaloupe, cherries, coconut, dates, figs, jujube (cooked), grapes, lemons, limes, mango, nectarines, oranges (sweet), papaya, peaches, pears, persimmons, plums (sweet), pomegranate, prunes, raspberries, raisins, strawberries
Small Amounts	Apples, bananas (sour), cranberries, grapefruit, pineapple (sweet), tangerines, watermelon
Avoid	Cherries, dry fruit, jujube (dry), pineapples (sour), plums (sour), oranges (sour), papaya, olives

Vegetables: Cooked vegetables are best as they are more
nourishing and easier to digest. Only leafy greens may be eaten raw
with dressing. More raw salads may be eaten in the hot summer if
digestion is strong and there is little gas or constipation.

Best	Artichoke (with oily dressing), avocado, bean sprouts, cauliflower, cilantro, corn, Jerusalem artichoke, leeks, okra, onion (cooked), peas, potato, pumpkin, seaweed, squash (acorn, winter, crook neck, zucchini etc.), sunflower sprouts, tomato (sweet vine ripened)
Small Amounts	Alfalfa sprouts, asparagus, beets, bell pepper, bitter melon, broccoli, brussel sprouts, cabbage, carrot, celery, cucumber, eggplant, green beans, lettuce (raw), kale, mushrooms, mustard greens, parsley, peas (sweet), spinach, sweet potato, tomato (sour), turnips
Avoid	Brussel sprouts, cabbage, chilies, hot peppers, radishes, raw onion, tomato paste and sauce, peas (snow)

Nuts and Seeds: These should be eaten lightly dry
roasted to assist digestion and only very lightly salted, if
at all. Nut butters, except for peanut, may also be eaten.

Best	Coconut, pinyon, sunflower seeds
Small Amounts	Almonds, Brazil nuts, cashews, lotus seeds, macadamia, pecans, pine, pistachio (non salted), pumpkin seeds
Avoid	Peanuts

Meats: Repeated research shows that plant based diets
are healthier than meat based diets and prevent many diseases.
Ayurveda and Yoga emphasize a vegetarian diet primarily for spiritual
reasons. Hence, omnivores should limit meat consumption if possible.
Weak patients should take them as a soup broth.

Meats: (cont'd)

Best	Chicken (white meat), egg, fresh water fish, pork, turkey (white meat)
Small Amounts	Duck, venison, beef, seafood, lamb
Avoid	Shell fish, dark meat of chicken or turkey

Legumes: Those listed in small amounts are best as a dal or spread with spices added. When digestion is weak or constipation present, even those beans listed under small amounts should be avoided.

Best	Mung beans, tofu
Small Amount	Aduki, black gram, chick peas, kidney, black lentils, navy, pinto, soy beans, split peas
Avoid	Fava, red and yellow lentils

Spices: Spices aid the digestion and absorption of nutrients as well as improve flavor. Food should have an overall spicing effect of being warming but not hot. It is the overall effect of spicing that is most important and not the individual spice used. Food should never be bland.

Best	Bay leaf, caraway, catnip, chamomile, cardamom, cilantro, cumin, coriander, dill, fennel, lemon verbena, peppermint, rose-mary, saffron, spearmint, turmeric
Small Amounts	Anise, basil, cinnamon, coconut, fenugreek, ginger (fresh), marjoram, nutmeg, oregano, poppy seeds, sage, salt, star anise, thyme
Avoid	Asafoetida, black pepper, cayenne, calamus, cloves, garlic (raw), ginger (dry), horseradish, hot mustards, hyssop

Condiments

Best	None
Small Amounts	Carob, mayonnaise
Avoid	Catsup, chocolate, tamari, vinegar

Beverages: These are best taken at room temperature or warm and never ice cold.

Best	Chamomile tea, licorice tea, mild spice teas, mint tea, milk, water
Small Amounts	Carrot juice (diluted), fruit juices (diluted), naturally flavored soda and juice beverages, tea (black or green)
Avoid	Alcohol, carrot juice (undiluted), coffee (caffeinated and decaffeinated), soft drinks and very spicy tea, sweet fruit juices (undiluted), tomato juice, vegetable juices (green)

2. VATA-KAPHA FOOD PROGRAM

BASIC PRINCIPLES

Qualities to reduce: Cold, dry and heavy
Best Taste: Pungent, sour
Small Amounts: Salty, astringent
Worst Tastes: Sweet, bitter

FOOD GROUPS

Grains: It is best to eat these as cooked grains, though a small amount of bread may be eaten.

Grains (cont'd)

Best	Amaranth, basmati Rice, barley, brown rice, quinoa, buckwheat, wild rice
Small Amounts	Millet, rye
Avoid	Corn flour, oats, rice (sticky, white, short or long grain), wheat

Dairy: It is best to use raw or organic milk products. Milk should be taken warm with a small amount of spices such as ginger and cardamom. Ghee and yogurt should also be used with warm spices.

Best	Two percent milk, buttermilk, ghee, low-fat yogurt
Small Amounts	Kefir, sour cream, yogurt (whole milk)
Avoid	Butter, cheeses, cottage cheese, ice cream, frozen yogurt, whole milk

Sweeteners: Overuse of any sweetener will eventually cause an imbalance. Those listed under small amounts are more likely to cause imbalances with regular usage and should not be used more than once each month.

Best	Honey
Small Amounts	Jaggery, molasses, sucanat
Avoid	Date sugar, dextrose, fructose, grape sugar, maltose, maple syrup, maple sugar, rice syrup, white table sugar

Oils: Oils are very important and should be used abundantly if the skin is dry. Though generally heavy, the lighter oils will not aggravate Kapha. Ghee should be used with warm spices.

Oils (cont'd)

Best	Flaxseed, ghee, mustard, safflower
Small Amounts	Almond, canola, castor, corn, margarine, olive, peanut, sesame, soy
Avoid	Avocado, coconut, soy, sunflower, lard

Fruit: Fruit is best when it is sour and not overly ripened or sweet. This will bring balance to both doshas. In general, due to its cooling effect on the body, fruit intake should be in small amounts. The best fruit may be taken in greater amounts. Fruit in general should not be a staple of the diet but is alright for occasional use.

Best	Apricots, cherries, grapefruit, lemon, papaya, pomegranate
Small Amounts	Apples (baked is best), banana (sour), blue-berries, blackberries, cranberries, cherries, lime, mango, oranges (sour), pineapple, plums (sour), pomegranate, prunes, rasp-berries, tangerines
Avoid	Avocado, banana (sweet), coconut, dates, figs, grapes (sweet), jujube, melons (water-melon, cantaloupe), oranges (sweet), peaches, nectar-ine, pears, persimmons, plums (sweet), raisins, strawberry

Vegetables: The diet should consist primarily of cooked vegetables. However, occasional use of raw vegetables is all right as long as there is no constipation or gas.

Best	Artichoke (with a spicy, oily dressing), beets, carrots, cauliflower, chili peppers, corn (whole, fresh), green beans, leeks, mung bean sprouts, mustard greens, onion, radish, parsley, potato, sunflower sprouts, tomato

Vegetables (cont'd)

Small Amounts	Alfalfa sprouts, avocado, bell peppers, broc-coli, brussel sprouts, celery, cilantro, kale, lettuce, mushrooms, okra, peas (green, snow), seaweed, spinach, swiss chard, ruta-bagas, squash (zucchini, crook neck), turnips
Avoid	Asparagus, bitter melon, cabbage, cucumber, eggplant, Jerusalem artichoke, squash (acorn, winter), sweet potato, yams

Nuts and Seeds: These should be taken lightly dry roasted to assist digestion and only very lightly salted, if at all. Nut butters, except for peanut, may also be eaten.

Best	Pumpkin seeds, sunflower seeds, pinyon
Small Amounts	Filberts
Avoid	Almonds, Brazil nuts, cashews, coconut, lotus seeds, macadamia, peanuts, pecans, pistachio, walnuts

Meats: Repeated research shows that plant based diets are healthier than meat based diets and prevent many diseases. Ayurveda and Yoga emphasize a vegetarian diet primarily for spiritual reasons. Hence, omnivores should limit meat consumption if possible. Weak patients should take meat as a soup broth.

Best	None
Small Amounts	Chicken and turkey (dark meat), salt water fish
Avoid	Beef, duck, pork, lamb, shell fish

Legumes: Legumes are best taken well cooked with warm spices as they can be hard to digest. Soaking them before cooking improves digestibility as well. As they contain earth and air, they are heavy and dry which can harm both doshas when digestion is weak. Those listed as best are easiest to digest and usually will not cause harm.

Legumes (cont'd)

Best	Mung beans, soy milk, tempeh, tofu
Small Amounts	None
Avoid	Aduki, black, black gram, chick peas, fava, kidney, lentils, lima, navy, peas (dry or split), pinto, soybeans

Spices: Spices aid the digestion and absorption of nutrients as well as improve flavor. Warm and hot spices are recommended for Vata-Kapha types. It is the overall effect of spicing that is most important and not the individual spice used. If food becomes too hot, it may contribute to greater dryness. Hence, the hottest spices should be used in moderation. Food should never be bland.

Best	Allspice, anise, asafoetida, basil, bay leaf, black pepper, caraway, catnip, cayenne, celery seed, chamomile, cloves, coriander, cumin, curry powder, dill, fennel, fenugreek, garlic, ginger, horseradish, hyssop, lemon verbena, marjoram, mustard seed, nutmeg, oregano, paprika, parsley, peppermint, poppy seed, rosemary, saffron, sage, star anise, spearmint, tarragon, thyme, turmeric
Small Amount	Salt
Avoid	None

Condiments

Best	Vinegar
Small Amounts	Catsup, carob (with proper sweeteners), chocolate (with proper sweeteners)
Avoid	Mayonnaise

Beverages: These are best taken at room temperature or warm and never ice cold.

Best	Water, chamomile tea, licorice tea, mint tea, spicy teas
Small Amounts	Vegetable juices, sour fruit juices (cranberry, lemon, lime, pineapple, pomegranate. Diluted preferred.)
Avoid	Black tea, coffee (caffeinated and decaf-feinated), alcohol, soft drinks, sweet fruit juices, sweetened soda pop

3. PITTA-KAPHA

BASIC PRINCIPLES

Qualities to reduce: Hot, heavy and moist
Best Taste: Bitter, astringent
Small Amounts: Pungent, sweet
Worst Tastes: Sour and salty

FOOD GROUPS

Grains: These may be eaten as cooked grains or as yeast breads.

Best	Barley, basmati rice, corn flour products (except corn chips), rye
Small Amounts	Amaranth, rice (brown), millet, quinoa
Avoid	Buckwheat, oats, wheat, white sticky rice

Dairy: It is best to use raw or organic milk products. Milk should be taken warm with a small amount of spices such as ginger and cardamom.

Best	Skim milk
Small Amounts	Ghee, goat milk, low-fat yogurt
Avoid	Butter, buttermilk, hard and soft cheeses, sour cream, cottage cheese, cream, frozen yogurt, kefir, ice cream, milk (whole), yogurt (whole milk)

Sweeteners: Overuse of any sweetener will eventually cause an imbalance.

Best	Stevia
Small Amounts	Fresh honey
Avoid	Brown sugar, date sugar, dextrose, fructose, grape sugar, honey (older than 6 months), maple syrup, maple sugar, maltose, rice syrup, molasses, white table sugar

Oils: Oils, being heavy and moist, should be generally used in small amounts in Pitta-Kapha types. The best oils are lighter, drier and cooler.

Best	Canola, corn, soy, sunflower
Small Amounts	Margarine, safflower
Avoid	Almond, avocado, castor, coconut, flaxseed, mustard, peanut, sesame, lard

Fruit: As fruit tends to be light and cooling, it is generally good for Pitta-Kapha types. Because it contains a lot of water, over use can aggravate Kapha. Dried fruit is the best though fresh fruit may be taken as well. Greater amounts may be eaten in the summer and less the rest of the year. Some sour fruits have the unique effect (prab-hava) of being cooling, despite the presence of fire in its taste. This makes it good for Pitta though it still may aggravate Kapha in excess.

Best	Apples, blueberries, cranberries, lemon, lime, pomegranate
Small Amounts	Apricots, blackberries, cantaloupe, cherries, grapefruit, jujube, watermelon, peaches, nectarines, oranges, pears, persimmons, pine-apple (sweet), plums (sweet), raspberries, tangerines
Avoid	Dates, figs, grapes, mango, papaya, pineapple (sour), sour plums, strawberries

Vegetables: Raw vegetables are best in the summer while a mixture of raw and cooked may be eaten the rest of the year. Light and cool, most vegetables reduce both Pitta and Kapha and thus should be eaten in great abundance.

Best	Alfalfa sprouts, artichokes, asparagus, bean sprouts, bell peppers, bitter melon, broccoli, brussel sprouts, cabbage, celery, cauliflower, cilantro, cooked onions, cress, eggplant, green beans, green peppers, kale, lettuce, leafy lettuce greens, mushrooms, peas (green, snow), pumpkin, parsley, sunflower sprouts, sweet peas, turnips
Small Amounts	Beets, corn, carrots, cucumber, cooked garlic, leeks, onion (fresh), parsley, potatoes, spinach, sweet tomatoes, mustard greens, okra, seaweed, spinach, squash (yellow)
Avoid	Avocado, chilies, eggplant, Jerusalem arti-choke, radish, onion(raw), tomato paste, squash (acorn, winter)

Nuts and Seeds: Heavy, oily and slightly warm, most nuts aggravate Pitta- Kapha individuals. Seeds are best, as they are lighter and drier.

Best	Pumpkin seeds, sunflower seeds
Small Amounts	Filberts, pinyon, sesame seeds
Avoid	Almonds, brazil, cashews, coconut, lotus seeds, macadamia, peanuts, pecans, pistachios, walnuts

Meats: Repeated research shows that plant based diets are healthier than meat based diets and prevent many diseases. Ayurveda and Yoga emphasize a vegetarian diet primarily for spiritual reasons. Hence, omnivores should limit meat consumption if possible. Weak patients should take meat as a soup broth. White meat is more balancing than dark meat

Best	None
Small Amounts	Chicken, egg (white), turkey, fresh water fish
Avoid	Beef, duck, egg (yolk), lamb, pork and sea-food, venison

Legumes: Beans tend to be dry, cool and somewhat heavy. Moderate use is generally alright for Pitta-Kapha types. They should be taken with spices to assist digestion. Soaking beans before cooking makes them easier to digest. Of all the beans, tofu and mung are the very best.

Best	Aduki, black gram, fava, kidney, lima, mung, navy, peas (split), pinto, soy beans and tofu
Small Amounts	Black beans
Avoid	Chick peas, lentils, peanuts, tempeh

Spices: Spices aid the digestion and absorption of nutrients as well as improve flavor. As Pitta-Kapha individuals generally feel warm, mild to moderate spicing is good. Care should be taken so that the overall

spiciness of the food is not too hot. It is the overall effect of spicing that is most important and not the individual spice used. Using large amounts of the best spices is recommended to enhance flavor.

Best	Cardamom, catnip, chamomile, coriander, cumin, curry leaves, fennel, lemon verbena, peppermint, saffron, spearmint, turmeric
Small Amounts	Allspice, anise, basil, bay leaves, caraway, dill, fenugreek, ginger (fresh), hyssop, ore-gano, paprika, parsley, poppy seeds, rose-mary, sage, star anise, tarragon, thyme
Avoid	Asafoetida, black pepper, calamus, cayenne pepper, celery seed, cinnamon, cloves, raw garlic, ginger (dry), horse radish, hot mus-tards, marjoram, nutmeg, salt

Condiments

Best	None
Small Amounts	Carob (sweetened with proper sweeteners)
Avoid	Catsup, chocolate, vinegar, mayonnaise

Beverages: These are best taken at room temperature or warm and never ice cold.

Best	Green vegetable juices, tea (chamomile, mint, spice teas from the spices "best" list), water with lemon
Small Amounts	Naturally carbonated pure juice drinks with no sugar added
Avoid	Black tea, coffee (caffeinated and decaf-fein-ated), alcohol, soft drinks, sweet fruit juices, sweetened soda pop, spicy teas

4. Tridoshic/Sannipatika Diet

BASIC PRINCIPLES

Qualities to reduce: Hot, heavy and dry
Best Taste: All in equal proportions

FOOD GROUPS

Grains: These may be eaten as cooked grains or as yeast breads.

Best	Basmati rice
Small Amounts	Amaranth, barley, brown rice, buckwheat, corn flour products, millet, quinoa
Avoid	None

Dairy: It is best to use raw or organic milk products. Milk should be taken warm with a small amount of spices such as ginger and cardamom. Ghee is best used with mild spices.

Best	Two percent milk, ghee
Small Amounts	Butter, buttermilk, sour cream, cottage cheese, cream, kefir, goat milk, whole cow's milk
Avoid	Hard cheese, ice cream, frozen yogurt

Sweeteners: Overuse of any sweetener will eventually cause an imbalance.

Best	Fresh honey
Small Amounts	Dextrose, date sugar, fructose, grape sugar, old honey, maple syrup, maple sugar, maltose, molasses, rice syrup, stevia
Avoid	White table sugar

Oils: The best oils are lighter, cooler and drier. They should be relied upon. Other oils may be used occasionally.

Best	Canola, corn, soy, sunflower
Small Amounts	Almond, avocado, castor, coconut, flaxseed, mustard, peanut, sesame, lard, margarine, safflower
Avoid	None

Fruit: Fruit tends to be light, cool and moist. Thus, it has the ideal qualities to bring balance to tridoshic individuals and can make up a significant portion of the diet. Those fruits listed under best, while not necessarily perfectly tridoshic, will not cause any serious imbalance if eaten regularly by tridoshic individuals.

Best	Apricots, apples, blackberries, blueberries, cantaloupe, cherries grapefruit, grapes, juju-be, lemon, lime, mango, nectarines, oranges, pears, watermelon, papaya, peaches, pears, plums pineapple, sweet plums, pomegranate, raspberries, tangerines
Small Amounts	Apples, bananas, cranberries, dates, figs, persimmons
Avoid	Cantaloupe, sour plums, strawberries

Vegetables: Vegetables are generally light, cool and dry. If cooked with water or oil, they become moist and slightly warmer. The best vegetables may be eaten regularly as a substantial part of the diet.

Best	Bean sprouts, cauliflower, cilantro, fresh corn, onions (cooked), leeks (cooked), parsley, potatoes, seaweed, sunflower sprouts

Vegetables (cont'd)

Small Amounts	Alfalfa sprouts, artichokes, asparagus, avo-cado, bell peppers, bitter melon, broccoli, brussel sprouts, cabbage, celery, cilantro, eggplant, green beans, green peppers, Jerusa-lem artichoke, kale, lettuce, mushrooms, peas, seaweed, okra, onion, sweet peas, turnips, green beans, pumpkin, cress, beets, corn, car-rots, cucumber, cooked garlic, leeks, mush-rooms, spinach, sweet tomatoes, mustard greens, okra, radish, seaweed, spinach, squash (yellow, acorn, winter)
Avoid	Hot chili peppers

Nuts and Seeds: Heavy, oily and slightly warm, most nuts will aggravate tridoshic individuals if relied upon as a staple. However, use in small amounts is advised and will not cause any imbalance.

Best	Pumpkin seeds, sunflower seeds, pinyon
Small Amounts	Almonds, brazil, cashews, coconut, filberts, lotus seeds, macadamia, peanuts, pecans, pistachio, sesame seeds, walnuts
Avoid	None

Meats: Repeated research shows that plant based diets are healthier than meat based diets and prevent many diseases. Ayurveda and Yoga emphasize a vegetarian diet primarily for spiritual reasons. Hence, omnivores should limit meat consumption if possible. Weak patients should take meat as a soup broth.

Best	None
Small Amounts	Beef, chicken, duck, egg, fish, lamb, pork, turkey
Avoid	None

Legumes: Beans tend to be dry, cool and somewhat heavy. Those listed under best are tridoshic. All beans should be taken with spices to assist digestion.

Best	Mung beans, tofu
Small Amounts	Aduki, black beans, black gram, chick peas, fava, kidney, lentils, lima, navy, peanuts, pinto beans, soy beans, tempeh
Avoid	None

Spices: Spices aid the digestion and absorption of nutrients as well as improve flavor. As tridoshic individuals generally feel warm, only moderate spicing is appropriate. Care should be taken so that the overall spiciness of the food is not too hot. It is the overall effect of spicing that is most important and not the individual spice used. Hence, even those listed under "avoid" may be used, but in the smallest amounts.

Best	Basil, bay leaves, chamomile, caraway, cardamom, catnip, coriander, cumin, dill, fennel, lemon verbena, peppermint, rose-mary, saffron, spearmint, turmeric
Small Amounts	Allspice, anise, asafetida, basil, bay leaves, black pepper, calamus, caraway, celery seed, cinnamon, curry leaves, dill, fenugreek, hy-ssop, marjoram, nutmeg, oregano, paprika, parsley, poppy seeds, rosemary, sage, salt, star anise, tarragon, thyme
Avoid	Cayenne pepper, cloves, raw garlic, dry ginger, horseradish, hot mustard

Condiments

Best	None
Small Amounts	Catsup, vinegar and mayonnaise
Avoid	None

Beverages: These are best taken at room temperature or warm and never ice cold.

Best	Water, water with lemon, herb teas with spices as listed
Small Amounts	Black tea, green vegetable juices, natural carbonated pure juice drinks
Avoid	Coffee (caffeinated and decaffeinated), alcohol, soft drinks, sweet fruit juices, sweetened soda pop

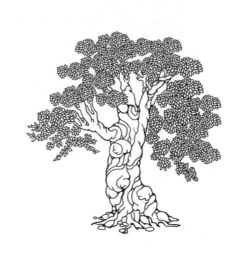

Glossary of Terms

Agni - fire, particularly the digestive fire

Ajña Chakra - center of command; third eye

Akasha - ether or space

Alochaka Pitta - form of Pitta governing vision

Ama - toxic material caused by poor digestion

Amla - sour taste

Ananda - bliss

Anna - food

Annamaya Kosha - food sheath

Annavaha Srotas - digestive system

Anuvasana Basti - oily enema

Apana Vayu - downward moving of the five breaths

Apas - the element of water

Arishta - herbal wine

Artava - menstrual fluid

Artavavaha Srotas - menstrual system

Artha - the goal of attaining wealth, resources or possessions

Asana - yoga posture

Asthi - bone

Ashtanga Hridaya - Ayurvedic text written by Vagbhatta

Atman - inner Self

Avalambaka Kapha - form of Kapha in the chest

Avaleha - herbal jelly

Avidya - ignorance

Ayurveda - the spiritual science of life (a supplement to the Vedas or Vedanga)

Bala - bodily strength

Basti - enema therapy (also means bladder)

Bahya Marga - outer disease pathway (skin and blood)

Bhakti Yoga - yoga of devotion

Bhrajaka Pitta - form of Pitta governing the complexion

Bhuta - element

Bhutagni - digestive fire governing an element

Bodhaka Kapha - form of Kapha giving sense of taste

Brahmacharya - control of sexual energy

Brimhana - tonification therapy

Buddhi - intelligence principle of discrimination

Chakra - spinal center of energy

Charaka - ancient Ayurvedic author

Charaka Samhita - Charaka's treatise on Ayurveda

Chikitsa - therapy (giving care to)

Daiva Chikitsa - spiritual therapy

Darshana - system of philosophy

Dharana - concentration, attention

Dharma - goal, principle, law of one's nature

Dhatu - tissue element of the body

Dhatvagni - Agni in the tissues

Dhyana - meditation

Dinacharya - daily regimen

Gati - quality of the pulse

Gunas - attributes, prime qualities of nature

Guru - quality of heaviness; spiritual teacher

Hatha Yoga - yoga of physical postures

Hridaya - heart

Japa - repetition of mantras

Jatharagni - digestive fire

Jiva - individual soul

Jñana Yoga - yoga of knowledge

Jyotish - Vedic Astrology

Kala - nutritional membrane for the tissues

Kama - desire

Kapha - biological water humor

Karma - bondage to action, the cause of rebirth

Karma Yoga - yoga of service

Kashaya - astringent taste

Katu - pungent or spicy taste

Kledaka Kapha - form of Kapha governing digestion

Kshatriya - man of political values

Kundalini - serpent fire

Laghu - lightness

Langhana - reducing therapy

Madhyama Marga - middle disease pathway (deep tissue)

Majja - bone marrow and nerve tissue

Mala - waste-material of the body

Mamsa - muscle

Manas - mind as principle of thought

Mantra - words of power, sacred sounds

Marana - Ayurvedic preparation of metals and minerals

Marga - pathway of the body

Marma - vital points on the body

Maya - illusion; cosmic creative power

Medas - fat

Moksha - liberation

Mutra - urine

Mutravaha Srotas - urinary system

Nadi - Ayurvedic name for pulse

Nadi pariksha - examination of pulse

Nasya - nasal administration of therapies

Nirama - condition of humors without products of indigestion

Niruha Basti - cleansing enema

Niyama - right actions or observances in yoga practice

Nyaya - one of the six Indian systems of philosophy

Ojas - primary energy reserve of body and mind

Pachaka Pitta - form of Pitta governing digestion

Pancha Karma - five cleansing actions of vomiting, purgation, enemas, bloodletting and nasal medications

Pariksha - examination or diagnosis

Patañjali - compiler of the classical Yoga system

Pitta - biological fire humor

Prabhava - special action of herbs

Prajñaparadha - failure of wisdom or intelligence

Prakriti - primal nature; natural state; constitution

Prakriti Pariksha - constitutional examination

Prana - life-force, breath, subtle form of the life-force, inward moving of the five breaths or life-force in the head

Pranayama - breath control

Prash - Ayurvedic herbal jelly

Pratyahara - control of senses and mind

Purisha - feces

Purishavaha Srotas - excretory system

Purusha - the original spirit, inner Self

Raga - attraction

Rajas - the intermediate principle of energy among the three qualities of nature (gunas)

Rajasic - having the nature of Rajas

Rakta - blood

Raktavaha Srotas - circulatory system (hemoglobin portion)

Rakta Moksha - therapeutic bloodletting

Rañjaka Pitta - form of Pitta coloring the blood

Rasa - plasma; taste

Rasayana - rejuvenation

Roga - disease

Ritucharya - seasonal regimen

Sadhaka Pitta - form of Pitta governing the brain

Sama - condition of humors with products of indigestion

Samana Vayu - equalizing form of the five breaths

Samkhya - the system of Indian philosophy enumerating the main principles of cosmic evolution used by all systems

Sattva - the higher principle of harmony of the three qualities of nature (gunas)

Sattvic - having the nature of Sattva

Satya - truth

Satya Buddhi - ascertainment of truth

Shakti - power, energy of consciousness

Shamana - palliation therapy

Shita - cool

Shiva - pure being or pure consciousness

Shodhana - purification therapy

Shukra - reproductive fluid

Shukravaha Srotas - reproductive system

Siddhi - psychic power

Sleshaka Kapha - form of

Kapha lubricating the joints

Sleshma - another name for Kapha or phlegm

Snehana - oleation therapy, oil massage

Sparshana - touch, palpation

Sushruta - ancient Ayurvedic author

Soma - bliss or pleasure principle at work behind the mind and senses

Srotas - the different channel systems or physiological systems

Sutra - axiom used in Vedic teaching

Swastha - health

Swasthya - state of being healthy

Swasthavritta - regimen promoting health

Swedana - sudation, steam or sweating therapy

Tail - medicated oil

Tamas - the lower principle of inertia of the three qualities of nature (gunas)

Tamasic - having the nature of Tamas

Tanmantra - five prime sensory principles (sound, touch, sight, taste and smell) behind organs and elements

Tantra - medieval yoga traditions emphasizing use of techniques and rituals

Tapas - discipline, self-discipline

Tarpaka Kapha - form of Kapha governing the brain and nerves

Tattva - principle of cosmic evolution (24 total)

Tejas - fire on a vital level

Tikta - bitter taste

Udana Vayu - upward moving of the five breaths

Upanishads - ancient Vedantic teachings of India

Ushna - hot

Vaidya - Ayurvedic doctor

Vagbhatta - ancient Ayurvedic author

Vajikarana - aphrodisiac

Vaisheshika - one of the six systems of Indian philosophy

Vamana - therapeutic vomiting

Vata - biological air humor

Vayas - life span

Vayu - another name for Vata

Vedas - ancient books of knowledge presenting the spiritual science of awareness

Vedanta - culmination of the Vedas in the philosophy of Self-realization

Vijñana - intelligence

Vikriti - disease state, diversification or deviation from nature

Vikriti pariksha - examination of disease

Vipaka - post-digestive effect of herbs

Virechana - purgation therapy

Virya - energetic effect of herbs as heating or cooling

Vishuddha Chakra - throat chakra

Vyana Vayu - outward moving of the five breaths

Yama - right attitudes in Yoga practice

Yoga - psychophysical practices aimed at Self-knowledge

Yoga Sutras - classical textbook of Yoga

Herb and Medicine Glossary

First listed is the common name of the herb used in the book, then the botanical name and the Ayurvedic name, if different from the common name.

Abhrak Bhasma - Ayurvedic oxide of mica

Aconite - Aconitum napellus, Visha

Agnimantha - Clerodendron phlomoides

Agrimony - Agrimonia eupatoria

Ajwan - Apium graveolens, Ajamoda

Aloe - Aloe spp. Kumari

Amalaki - Emblica officinalis

Anu Tail - Type of medicated sesame oil

Apamarga - Achyranthes aspera

Aragwadha - Cassia fistula

Arjuna - Terminalia arjuna

Asafoetida - Ferula asafoetida, Hingu

Ashok - Saraca indica

Ashwagandha - Withania somnifera

Ashwatta - Ficus religiosa

Ativisha - Aconitum heterophyllum

Bakuchi - Psoralea corylifolia

Bala - Sida cordifolia

Barberry - Berberis spp., Daruharidra

Bayberry - Myrica spp., Katphala

Bhallataka - Semecarpus anacardium

Bhringaraj - Eclipta alba

Bhumyamalaki - Pyllanthus niruri

Bibhitaki - Terminalia belerica

Bilwa - Aegle marmelos

Black Pepper - Piper nigrum, Marich

Brahma Rasayan - herbal jelly mainly consisting of brahmi or gotu kola

Brahmi - Hydrocotyle asiatica or Bacopa monnieri (preferable herb)

Brahmi Oil - Medicated coconut oil prepared mainly with gotu kola

Brihati - Solanum indicum

Calamus - Acorus calamus, Vacha

Camphor - Cinnamomum camphora, Karpura

Cardamom - Elettaria cardamomum, Ela

Castor oil - Ricinis communis, Eranda

Catechu - Acacia catechu, Khadir

Cayenne - Capsicum frutescens, Katuvira

Chandanbalalakshadi Tail - cooling, medicated oil consisting mainly of sandalwood and bala

Chandraprabha - special Ayurvedic formula for weak kidneys

Chavya - Piper chaba

Chiretta - Swertia chirata, Kiratatikta

Chitrak - Plumbago zeylonica

Chyavan Prash - Herbal jelly (prash) mainly consisting of amalaki fruit

Cinnamon - Cinnamomum zeylonica, Twak

Cinnamon leaf -Cinnamomum tamala, Tejapatra

Citron - Citrus Bijapura

Cloves - Syzgium aromaticum, Lavanga

Coral Ash - Ayurvedic coral preparation, Prawal Bhasma

Coriander - Coriandrum sativum, Dhanyaka

Cubebs - Piper cubeba, Kankola

Cumin - Cumin cyminum, Jiraka

Cuscuta - Cuscuta reflexa, Amaravalli

Cyperus - Cyperus rotundus, Musta

Dandelion - Taraxacum vulgare, Dughdapheni

Darbha - Imperatu cylindrica

Datura - Datura alba, Kanaka-dattura

Dill - Anthemum vulgaris, Mishreya

Dhataki - Woodfordia floribunda

Draksha - Ayurvedic herbal grape wine

Echinacea - Echinacea angustifolia

Elecampane - Inula spp., Pushkaramula

Emetic Nut - Randia dumetorum, Madana-phala

Ephedra - Ephedra spp., Somalata

Eucalyptus - Eucalyptus globulis, Tailaparni

Fennel - Foeniculum vulgare, Shatapushpa

Fenugreek - Trigonella foenum-graecum, Methi

Flaxseed - Linum usitatissimum, Uma

Gambhari - Gmelina arborea

Garlic - Allium sativum, Lashuna

Gentian - Gentiana spp., Trayamana

Ginger - Zingiberis officinalis, Ardra (fresh), Shunthi (dry)

Ginseng - Panax ginseng, Lakshmana

Gokshura - Tribulis terrestris

Gold Bhasma - Special Ayurvedic mineral preparation made with gold Suvarna Bhasma

Golden seal - Hydrastis canadensis

Gotu kola - Centella or Hydrocotyle asiatica

Guduchi - Tinospora cordifolia

Guggul - Commiphora mukul (made with other herbs into various resin preparations called Gugguls)

Gurmar - Gymena sylvestre, Meshashringi

Harenu - Vitex agnus-castus

Haritaki - Terminalia chebula

Holy Basil - Ocimum sanctum, Tulsi

Jambu - Eugenia jambolana

Jasmine - Jasminum grandiflorum, Jati

Jatamamsi - Nardostachys jatamamsi

Jivanti - Dendrobium macrael

Kakoli - Polygonatum verticillatum

Kalajaji - Eugenia jambolanum

Kantakari - Solanum xanthocarpum

Kapittha - Feronia elephantum

Kapikacchu - Mucuna pruriens

Karanj - Pongomia glabra

Kasa - Saccharum spontaneum

Katuka - Picrorrhiza kurroa

Kokilaksha - Asteracantha longifolia

Kukkutanda Bhasma - Oxide made from peacock feathers

Kumbhi - Cares arborea

Kusha - Desmostachya bipinnata

Kushta - Saussurea lappa

Kutaj - Holarrhena antidysenterica

Lauhadi Rasayana - Rejuvenative medicine made mainly with iron

Lemon grass - Cymbopogon citratus, Rohisha

Licorice - Glycyzrrhiza spp., Yashtimadhu

Lodhra - Symplocus racemosus

Loha Bhasma - Specially prepared iron ash

Long Pepper - Piper longum, Pippali

Lotus - Nelumbo nucifera, Padma

Mahabala - Sida rhombifolia

Makaradhwaj - Ayurvedic alchemical compound consisting of purified sulphur and mercury along with herbs like camphor nutmeg cloves and Trikatu

Mandukaparni - Brahmi substitute

Manjishta - Rubia cordifolium

Masha - Phaseolus roxburghii

Meda - Rosocoea alpinia

Mrigashringa - Bhasma Ash or oxide made from deer horn

Mustard - Brassica alba, Shwetarisha

Myrrh - Commiphora myrrha, Bola

Nagakeshar - Mesua ferrea

Nagbala - Sida spinosa

Narayan Tail - Medicated sesame oil made mainly with shatavari

Neem - Azadiracta indica, Nimbu

Nirgundi - Vitex negundo

Nishot - Ipomoea turpethum

Nutmeg - Myristica fragrans, Jatiphala

Nux vomica - Strychnos nux-vomica

Nyagrodha - Ficus bengalensis

Parisha - Hibiscus populnea

Pashana bheda - Bergenia ligulata

Patala - Stereospermum suaveolens

Patola - Trichosanthes cucumerina

Pennyroyal - Mentha pulegium

Peppermint - Mentha piperata, Phudina

Pinus roxurghii - Sarala

Plaksha - Ficus infectoria

Pomegranate - Punica granatum, Dadima

Prishniparni - Uraria picta

Priyangu - Prunus mahaleb

Psyllium - Plantago psyllium, Snigdhajira

Prasarini - Paedaria foetida

Punarnava - Boerrhavia diffusa

Rasna - Pluchea lanceolata

Rhubarb root - Rheum spp., Amlavetasa

Rohitak - Tecomella undulata

Saffron - Crocus sativa, Keshar

Sandalwood - Santalum alba, Chandana

Sarsaparilla - Smilax spp., Chopchini

Saussurea - Saussurea lappa, Kushta

Senna - Cassia acutifolia, Nripadruma

Shalaparni - Desmodium gangetum

Shallaki - Boswellia serrata

Shankhapushpi - Crotalaria verrucosa

Shatavari - Asparagus racemosus

Shigru - Moringa concanensis

Shikai - Acacia concina

Shilajit - Asphaltum

Shinshipa - Dalbergia latifolia

Shirisha - Albizzia lebbek

Shukti Bhasma - Special Ayurvedic mineral preparation made from mother of pearl

Shyonaka - Oroxylum indicum

Silver Bhasma - Rajata Bhasma

Simhanad Guggul - Guggul made with triphala, sulphur and castor oil

Sitopaladi churna - Ayurvedic powder consisting of raw sugar, vamsharochana, long pepper and cinnamon

Soapnut tree - Sapindus trifoliatus

Suvarna makshika - Ayurvedic chalkopyrite preparation, a compound of copper, iron and sulphur

Suvarna parpatti -

Ayurvedic gold preparation

Trikatu - Ayurvedic formula consisting of dry ginger, black pepper and long pepper (pippali)

Triphala - Ayurvedic formula consisting of haritaki, amalaki and bibhitaki

Triphala guggul - Medicated resin or guggul made with the formula triphala

Trivrit - Ipomoea turpethum

Turmeric - Curcuma longa, Haridra

Tuverak - Hydnocarpus laurifolia

Udumbara - Ficus glomerata

Valerian - Valeriana spp., Tagara

Vateria indica - Ajakarna

Vetivert - Andropogon muricatus, Ushira

Vetra - Salix caprea

Violet - Viola spp., Banafshah

Vamsharochana - Bambusa arundinacea

Vidanga - Embelia ribes

Vidari - Pueraria tuberosa

White musali - Asparagus adscendens Shveta musali

Wintergreen - Gaultheria procumbens Gandapura

Yavani - Trachyspermum ammi

Yogaraj Guggul - Guggul formula particularly useful for arthritis

Bibliography

Charaka. Charaka Samhita. Varanasi, India: Chowkhamba Sanskrit Series, 1976.

Dash, Bhagavan. Concept of Agni in Ayurveda. Varanasi India: Chowkhamba Sanskrit Series, 1971.

Dash, Bhagavan and Manfred Junius. A Handbook of Ayurveda. New Delhi, India: Concept Publishing, 1983.

Dwarakanath, Dr. C.D. Introduction to Kayachikitsa. Varanasi, India: Chaukhambha Orientalia, 1986.

Frawley. Dr. David. Ayurveda and the Mind. Twin Lakes, Wisconsin: Lotus Press, 1997.

Frawley, Dr. David. Ayurvedic Healing: A Comprehensive Guide. Twin Lakes, Wisconsin: Lotus Press, 2000.

Frawley. Dr. David. Yoga and Ayurveda. Twin Lakes, Wisconsin: Lotus Press, 1999.

Frawley, Dr. David and Dr. Vasant Lad. The Yoga of Herbs. Santa Fe, New Mexico: Lotus Press, 1986.

Joshi, Dr. Sunil. Ayurveda and Pancha Karma. Twin Lakes, Wisconsin: Lotus Press 1997.

Lad, Dr. Vasant. Ayurveda, The Science of Self-healing. Santa Fe, New Mexico: Lotus Press, 1984.

Lad, Dr. Vasant. The Complete Book of Ayurvedic Home Remedies. New York City: Harmony Books, 1998.

Lele, Dr. R.D. Ayurveda and Modern Medicine. Bombay, India: Bharatiya Vidya Bhavan, 1986.

Morningstar, Amadea. The Ayurvedic Cookbook. Twin Lakes, Wisconsin: Lotus Press, 1992.

Morningstar, Amadea. Ayurvedic Cooking for Westerners. Twin Lakes, Wisconsin: Lotus Press, 1996.

Nadkarni. Indian Materia Medica. Bombay, India: Popular Prakashan, 1976.

Savnur, H.V. Ayurvedic Materia Medica. Delhi, India: Indian Books Centre, 1984.

Smith, Atreya. Ayurvedic Healing for Women. York Beach, Maine: Samuel Weiser, 1999.

Smith, Atreya. Practical Ayurveda. York Beach, Maine: Samuel Weiser, 1997.

Sushruta. Sushruta Samhita. Varanasi India: Chowkhamba Sanskrit Series, 1981.

Tarabilda, Ed. Ayurveda Revolutionized. Twin Lakes, Wisconsin, Lotus Press, 1998.

Thakur, C.G. Ayurveda the Indian Art and Science of Medicine. New York, New York: C.G.A.S.I. Publications, 1981.

Tierra, Michael. Planetary Herbology. Santa Fe, New Mexico: Lotus Press, 1988.

Udupa, K.N. and R.H. Singh. Science and Philosophy of Indian Medicine. Nagpur, India: Shree Baidyanath Ayurved Bhawan Ltd., 1978.

Vagbhatta. Ashtanga Hridaya. (Sanskrit only)

Resources

American Institute of Vedic Studies

The American Institute of Vedic Studies is an educational center devoted to the greater systems of Vedic and Yogic knowledge. It teaches various related aspects of Vedic Science including Ayurveda, Vedic Astrology, Yoga, Tantra and Vedanta with special reference to their background in the Vedas. The Institute is also engaged in many educational projects in the greater field of Hindu Dharma. Long term Institute research projects include:

- Ayurvedic Psychology and Yoga: The mental and spiritual aspect of Ayurveda relative to Raja Yoga and Vedanta.
- Medical Astrology: Relative to both health and disease for body and mind.
- Translations and interpretations of the Vedas, particularly the Rig Veda, and an explication of the original Vedic Yoga.
- Vedic History: The history of India and of the world from a Vedic perspective and also as reflecting latest archaeological work in India.
- Vedic Europe: Explaining the connections between the Vedic and ancient European cultures and religions.
- Projection of Vedic and Hindu knowledge in a modern context for the coming millennium.

The Institute has helped found various organizations including the New England Institute of Ayurvedic Medicine, the California College of Ayurveda, the American Council of Vedic Astrology, the World Association for Vedic Studies, and the British Association of Vedic Astrology.

American Institute of Vedic Studies
PO Box 8357, Santa Fe NM 87504-8357
Ph: 505-983-9385, Fax: 505-982-5807
David Frawley (Vamadeva Shastri), Director
Web: www.vedanet.com, Email: vedicinst@aol.com

American Institute of Vedic Studies
Ayurvedic Healing Correspondence Course

This comprehensive practical program covers all the main aspects of Ayurvedic theory, diagnosis and practice, with special emphasis on herbal medicine and on dietary therapy. It also goes in detail into Yoga philosophy and Ayurvedic psychology, showing an integral approach of mind-body medicine. It contains all the material covered in two-year Ayurvedic programs for foreign students in India.

The course is designed for Health Care Professionals as well as serious students to provide the foundation for becoming an Ayurvedic practitioner. It has been taken by doctors, chiropractors, nurses, acupuncturists, herbalists, massage therapists, yoga therapists and psychologists. However, there is no required medical background for those wishing to take the course and many non-professionals have completed it successfully. Topics include: Ayurvedic Anatomy and Physiology, Determination of Constitution, Diagnosis, the Disease Process, Samkhya and Yoga, Diet and Nutrition, Ayurvedic Herbology, Aroma Therapy, Ayurvedic Psychology, Mantra and Meditation, and more.

Since 1988, over two thousand people have taken the course, which is the most comprehensive correspondence course on this subject offered in the West. It is also the basis for Ayurvedic programs taught in the United States, UK, Europe, Australia and India.

The course is authored by Dr. David Frawley (Pandit Vamadeva Shastri), uses his books on Ayurveda, and represents his approach to Ayurveda, adapting Ayurveda to the modern world without losing its spiritual integrity.

American Institute Of Vedic Studies
Astrology of the Seers Correspondence Course

This comprehensive homestudy course explains Vedic Astrology in clear and modern terms, providing practical insights on how to use and adapt the system. For those who have difficulty approaching the Vedic system, the course provides many keys for unlocking its language and its methodology for the Western student.

The goal of the course is to provide the foundation for the student to become a professional Vedic astrologer. The orientation of the course is twofold: To teach the language, approach and way of thinking of Vedic Astrology and to teach the Astrology of Healing of the Vedic system, or Ayurvedic Astrology. Topics include: Planets, Signs, Houses, Aspects, Yogas, Nakshatras, Dashas, Divisional Charts, Ashtakavarga, Muhurta, Ayurvedic Astrology, Spiritual Astrology, Gemtherapy, Mantras and Deities, and Principles of Chart Analysis.

The course can be taken as part of a longer tutorial program of training in Vedic Astrology through the American Council of Vedic Astrology (ACVA), the largest Vedic Astrology organization outside of India, and counts for two hundred of the total six hundred credit hours for the program.

International Academy of Ayurveda

The International Academy of Ayurveda in Pune, India is one of the foremost institutions for training foreign students in India. It has complete facilities and programs for all levels of training from beginner to advanced, including special clinical instruction. It features a renowned faculty of Ayurvedic experts from throughout the world including Dr. Subhash Ranade, Dr. Avinash Lele, Dr. Abbas Qutab, Dr. Marc Halpern, Dr. Hans Rhyner, Dr. David Frawley, and Mukunda Stiles. Pune itself is one of the most modern cities in India with a pleasant year round climate and easy airport access from Bombay (Mumbai), making it an ideal place in India to study.

The Institute offers practical courses in Ayurveda, both Basic and Advanced. Special programs are available on the Fundamentals of Ayurveda, Panchakarma, Ayurvedic Massage, Marma Therapy, Herbology and Clinical Studies. Programs are given July-August and November-January every year in batches of about ten students. Please register at least two months ahead of time to reserve your place.

The Institute has its own line of a dozen important books on Ayurveda in English by Dr. Ranade, Dr. Lele, Dr. Frawley, and others, as well as other educational materials (Ayurvedic CD-ROM) and herbal products.

International Academy of Ayurveda
Nand Nandan, Atreya Rugnalaya, M.Y. Lele Chowk
Erandawana, Pune 411 004 India
Telefax 91-11-212-378532/ 524427
www.ayurveda-int.com

Aromatherapy Study Programs

Quintessence Aromatherapy
Attn: Ann Berwick
P. O. Box 4996
Boulder, CO 80306
Ph: 303-258-3791

Ayurveda Centers and Programs

Australian Institute of
Ayurvedic Medicine
19 Bowey Avenue
Enfield S.A. 5085
Australia
Ph: 08-349-7303

Australian School of Ayurveda
Dr. Krishna Kumar, MD, FIIM
27 Blight Street
Ridleyton, South Australia 5008
Ph. 08-346-0631

Ayur-Veda AB
Box 78, 285 22 Markaryd
Esplanaden 2
Sweden
0433-104 90 (Phone)
0433-104 92 (Fax)
E-mail: info@ayur-veda.se

Ayurveda for Radiant Health &
Beauty
16 Espira Court
Santa Fe, NM 87505
Ph: 505-466-7662

Ayurvedic HealingArts Center
16508 Pine Knoll Road
Grass Valley, CA 95945
Ph: 916-274-9000

Ayurvedic Healings
Dr's Light & Bryan Miller

P. O. Box 35214
Sarasota, FL 34242
Ph: 941-346-3581

Ayurvedic Holistic Center
82A Bayville Ave.
Bayville, NY 11709

The Ayurvedic Institute and
Wellness Center
11311 Menaul, NE
Albuquerque, NM 87112
Ph: 505-291-9698
Fax: 505-294-7572

Ayurvedic LivingWorkshops
P. O. Box 188
Exeter, Devon EX4 5AB
England

California College of Ayurveda
1117A East Main Street
Grass Valley, CA 95945
Ph: 530-274-9100
Website: ayurvedacollege.com
E-mail: info@ayurvedacollege.
com
Clinical training in Ayurveda

Center for Mind, Body
Medicine
P. O. Box 1048
La Jolla, CA 92038
Ph: 619-794-2425

The Chopra Center for
Well-Being
7630 Fay Ave.
LaJolla, CA 92037
Ph: 858-551-7788
888-424-6772

John Douillard
Life Spa, Rejuvenation through
Ayur-Veda
3065 Center Green Dr.

Boulder, CO 80301
Ph: 303-442-1164
Fax: 303-442-1240

East West College of Herbalism
Ayurvedic Program
Represents courses of Dr. David
Frawley and Dr. Michael Tierra
in UK
Hartswood, Marsh Green,
Hartsfield
E. Sussex TN7 4ET
United Kingdom
Ph: 01342-822312
Fax: 01342-826346
E-mail: ewcolherb@aol.com

Himalayan Institute
RR1, Box 400
Honesdale, PA 18431
Ph: 800-822-4547
E-mail: earthess@aol.com
Website: ayurvedichealing.com

Institute for Wholistic
Education
3425 Patzke Lane,
Racine, WI 53405
Ph: 262-619-1798
Beginner and Advanced
Correspondence Courses in
Ayurveda.

Integrated Health Systems
3855 Via Nova Marie, #302D
Carmel, CA 93923
Ph: 408-476-5130

International Academy of
Ayurved
NandNandan, Atreya Rugna-
laya
M.Y. Lele Chowk
Erandawana, Pune
411 004, India

Ph/Fax: 91-212-378532/524427
E-mail: avilele@hotmail.com

International Ayurvedic Insti-
tute
111 Elm St., Ste. 103-105
Worcester, MA 01609
Ph: 508-755-3744
Fax: 508-770-0618
E-mail: ayurveda@hotmail.com

International Federation of
Ayurveda
Dr. Krishna Kumar
27 Blight Street
Ridleyton S.A. 5008
Australia
Ph: 08-346-0631

Kaya Kalpa International
Dr. Raam Panday
111 Woodster Rd.
Satto, NY 10012

Life Impressions Institute
Attn: Donald VanHowten,
Director
613 Kathryn Street
Santa Fe, NM 87501
Ph: 505-988-2627

Light Institute of Ayurveda
Dr's Bryan & Light Miller
P. O. Box 35284
Sarasota, FL 34242
E-mail: earthess@aol.com
Website: ayurvedichealings.com

Lotus Ayurvedic Center
4145 Clares St., Ste. D
Capitola, CA 95010
Ph: 408-479-1667

Lotus Press
P. O. Box 325
Twin Lakes, WI 53181 USA

800-824-6396 (toll free order line)
Ph: 262-889-8561
Fax: 262-889-8591
E-mail: lotuspress@lotuspress.com
Website: www.lotuspress.com
Publisher of books on Ayurveda, Reiki, aromatherapy, energetic healing, herbalism, alternative health and U.S. editions of Sri Aurobindo's writings.

Maharishi Ayurved at the Raj
1734 Jasmine Avenue
Fairfield, IA 52556
Ph: 800-248-9050
Fax: 515-472-2496

Maharishi Health Center
Hale Clinic
7 Park Crescent
London, W14 3H3
England

Natural Therapeutics Center
Surya Daya
Gisingham, Nr. Iye
Suffolk, England

Rocky Mountain Ayurveda
Health Retreat
P. O. Box 5192
Pagosa Springs, CO 81147
Ph: 800-247-9654; 970-264-9224

Atreya Smith, Director
European Institute of Vedic Studies
Ceven Point N° 230
4 bis rue Taisson
30100 Ales, France
Fax: 33-466-60-53-72
E-mail: atreya@compuserve.com

Website: www.atreya.com

Vinayak Ayurveda Center
2509 Virginia NE, Suite D
Albuquerque, NM 87110
Ph: 505-296-6522
Fax: 505-298-2932
Website: www.ayur.com

Wise Earth School of Ayurveda
Attn: Bri. Maya Tiwari
90 Davis Creek Road
Candler, NC 28715
Ph: 828-258-9999
Fax: 828-667-0844
Teachers and Practitioners
Training Programs Only.

Ayurvedic Cosmetic Companies

Auroma International
1100 Lotus Light Dr
Silver Lake, WI 53170 USA
Ph: 262-889-8569
Fax: 262-889 8591
E-mail: auroma@lotuspress.com
Website: www.auroma.net
Importer and master distributor of Auroshikha Incense, Chandrika Ayurvedic Soap and Herbal Vedic Ayurvedic products.

Bindi Facial Skin Care
A Division of Pratima Inc.
109-17 72nd Road
Lower Level
Forest Hills, New York 11375
Ph: 718-268-7348

Devi Inc. (for Shivani product line)
Attn: Anjali Mahaldar

P. O. Box 377
Lancaster, MA 01523
Ph: 800-237-8221
Fax: 508-368-0455

Internatural
P O Box 489
Twin Lakes, WI. 53181 USA
800-643 4221 (toll free order
line)
262-889 8581 (office phone)
262-889 8591 (fax)
E-mail:
internatural@lotuspress.com
Website: www.internatural.com
Retail mail order and internet
reseller of Ayurvedic products,
essential oils, herbs, spices,
supplements, herbal remedies,
incense, books and other supplies.

Lotus Brands, Inc.
1100 Lotus Light Dr
Silver Lake, WI 53170 USA
Ph: 262-889-8561
Fax: 262-889-8591
E-mail:
lotusbrands@lotuspress.com
Website:
www.lotusbrands.com
Manufacturer and distributor of
natural personal care and herbal
products, massage oils, essential
oils, incense, aromatherapy
items, dietary supplements and
herbs.

Lotus Light Enterprises
1100 Lotus Drive
Silver Lake, WI 53170 USA
800-548 3824 (toll free order
line)

262-889 8501 (office phone)
262-889 8591 (fax)
E-mail:
lotuslight@lotuspress.com
Website: www.lotuslight.com
Wholesale distributor of essential oils, herbs, spices, supplements, herbal remedies, incense, books and other supplies.
Must supply resale certificate
number or practitioner license
to obtain catalog of more than
10,000 items.

Siddhi Ayurvedic Beauty Prod-
ucts
C/O Vinayak Ayurveda Center
2509 Virginia NE, Suite D
Albuquerque, NM 87110
Ph: 505-296-6522
Fax: 505-298-2932

Swami Sada Shiva Tirtha
Ayurvedic Holistic Center
82A Bayville Avenue
Bayville, NY 11709
Ph/Fax: 516-628-8200

TEJ Beauty Enterprises, Inc.
(an AyurvedicBeauty Salon)
162 West 56th St. Rm 201
New York, NY 10019
(owner: Pratima Raichur,
founder of Bindi)
Ph: 212-581-8136

Ayurvedic Herbal Suppliers

Auroma International
1100 Lotus Light Dr
Silver Lake, WI 53170 USA

Ph: 262-889-8569
Fax: 262-889 8591
E-mail:
auroma@lotuspress.com
Website: www.auroma.net
Importer and master distributor of Auroshikha Incense, Chandrika Ayurvedic Soap and Herbal Vedic Ayurvedic products.

Ayur Herbal Corporation
P. O. Box 6390
Santa Fe, NM 87502
Ph: 262-889-8569
Manufacturer of Herbal Vedic Ayurvedic products.

Ayush Herbs, Inc.
10025 N.E. 4th Street
Bellevue, WA 98004
Ph: 800-925-1371

Banyan Trading Company
Traditional Ayurvedic Herbs - Wholesale
P. O. Box 13002
Albuquerque, NM 87192
Ph: 505-244-1880; 800-953-6424
Fax: 505-244-1878

Bazaar of India Imports, Inc.
1810 University Avenue
Berkeley, CA 94703
Ph: 800-261-7662; 510-548-4110

Dhanvantri Aushadhalaya
Herbs of Wisdom and Love, Ayurvedic Herbs and Classical Formulas.
P. O. Box 1654
San Anselmo, CA 94979
Ph: 415-289-7976
Email:
ayurveda@dhanvantri.com

Dr. Singha's Mustard Bath and More
Attn: Anna Searles
Natural Therapeutic Centre
2500 Side Cove
Austin, TX 78704
Ph: 800-856-2862

Bio Veda
215 North Route 303
Congers, NY 10920-1726
Ph: 800-292-6002

Earth Essentials Florida
Dr's Bryan and Light Miller
4067 Shell Road
Sarasota, FL 34242
Ph: 941-316-0920

Frontier Herbs
P. O. Box 229
Norway, IA 52318
Ph: 800-669-3275

HerbalVedic Products
P. O. Box 6390
Santa Fe, NM 87502

Internatural
P O Box 489
Twin Lakes, WI. 53181 USA
800-643-4221 (toll free order line)
262-889-8581 (office phone)
262-889-8591 (fax)
E-mail:
internatural@lotuspress.com
Website: www.internatural.com
Retail mail order and internet reseller of Ayurvedic products, essential oils, herbs, spices, supplements, herbal remedies, incense, books and other supplies.

Lotus Brands, Inc.
1100 Lotus Light Dr
Silver Lake, WI 53170 USA
Ph: 262-889-8561
Fax: 262-889-8591
E-mail:
lotusbrands@lotuspress.com
Website:
www.lotusbrands.com

Lotus Herbs
1505 42nd Ave., Suite 19
Capitola, CA 95010
Ph: 408-479-1667

Lotus Light Enterprises
1100 Lotus Drive
Silver Lake, WI 53170 USA
800-548-3824 (toll free order line)
262-889-8501 (office phone)
262-889-8591 (fax)
E-mail:
lotuslight@lotuspress.com
Website: www.lotuslight.com
Wholesale distributor of
Ayurvedic products, essential
oils, herbs, spices, supplements,
herbal remedies, incense, books
and other supplies. Must supply resale certificate number or
practitioner license to obtain
catalog of more than 10,000
items.

Maharishi Ayurveda Products
International, Inc.
417 Bolton Road
P. O. Box 541
Lancaster, MA 01523
Info: 800-843-8332 Ext. 903
Order: 800-255-8332 Ext. 903

Planetary Formulations
P. O. Box 533
Soquel, CA 95073
Formulas by Dr. Michael Tierra

Quantum Publication, Inc.
P. O. Box 1088
Sudbury, MA 01776
Ph: 800-858-1808

Seeds of Change
P. O. Box 15700
Santa Fe, NM 87506-5700
Catalog of rare Western and
Indian seeds.

Vinayak Panchakarma Chikit-salaya
Y.M.C.A Complex, Situbuldi
Nagpur (Maharastra State)
India 440 012
Ph: 011-91-712-538983
Fax: 011-91-712-552409
Retail/Wholesale

Yoga of Life Center
2726 Tramway N.E.
Albuquerque, NM 87122
Ph: 505-275-6141

The Center For Release and
Integration
450 Hillside Drive
Mill Valley, CA 94941

Dr. Jay Scherer's Academy of
Natural Healing
1443 St. Francis Drive
Santa Fe, NM 87505

The Rolf Institute
205 Canyon Blvd.
Boulder, CO 80302

The Upledger Institute
1211 Prosperity Farms Rd.
Palm Beach Gardens, FL 33410

Correspondence Courses

American Institute of Vedic Studies
Dr. David Frawley, Director
P. O. Box 8357
Santa Fe, NM 87504-8357
Ph: 505-983-9385
Fax: 505-982-5807
E-mail: vedicinst@aol.com
Website: www.vedanet.com
Correspondence courses in Ayurveda and Vedic Astrology

Light Institute of Ayurvedic Teaching
Dr's Bryan & Light Miller
P. O. Box 35284Sarasota, FL 34242
Ph: 941-346-3518
Fax: 941-346-0800
E-mail: earthess@aol.com
Website:
www.ayurvedichealing.com
Ayurvedic Pratitioner Training, Correspondence Course, Books

Lessons and Lectures in Ayurveda by Dr. Robert Svoboda
P. O. Box 23445
Albuquerque, NM 87192-1445
Ph: 505-291-9698

Institute for Wholistic Education
3425 Patzke Lane,
Racine, WI 53405 USA
Ph: 262-619-1798
Beginner and Advanced Correspondence Courses in Ayurveda.

To train in Ayurvedic Facial Massage and Beauty practices

Melanie Sachs
"Invoking Beauty with Ayurveda" Seminars
P. O. Box 13753
San Luis Obispo, CA 93406

Beauty and Quality Ayurvedic Supplements

Auroma International
1100 Lotus Light Dr
Silver Lake, WI 53170 USA
Ph: 262-889-8569
Fax: 262- 889 8591
E-mail:
auroma@lotuspress.com
Website: www.auroma.net
Importer and master distributor of Auroshikha Incense, Chandrika Ayurvedic Soap and Herbal Vedic Ayurvedic products.

Ayur Herbal Corporation
P. O. Box 6390 AN
Santa Fe, NM 87502
Ph: 262-889-8569
Fax: 262-889 8591
Manufacturer of Herbal Vedic Ayurvedic products.

Internatural
P O Box 489
Twin Lakes, WI. 53181 USA
800-643-4221 (toll free order line)
262-889-8581 (office phone)
262-889 8591 (fax)
E-mail:

internatural@lotuspress.com
Website: www.internatural.com
Retail mail order and internet
reseller of Ayurvedic products,
essential oils, herbs, spices,
supplements, herbal remedies,
incense, books and other supplies.

Lotus Brands, Inc.
1100 Lotus Light Dr
Silver Lake, WI 53170 USA
Ph: 262-889-8561
Fax: 262-889-8591
E-mail:
lotusbrands@lotuspress.com
Website: www.lotuspress.com
Manufacturer and distributor of
natural personal care and herbal
products, massage oils, essential
oils, incense and aromatherapy
items.

Lotus Light Enterprises
1100 Lotus Drive
Silver Lake, WI 53170 USA
800-548-3824 (toll free order
line)
262-889-8501 (office phone)
262-889-8591 (fax)
E-mail:
lotuslight@lotuspress.com
Website: www.lotuslight.com
Wholesale distributor of
Ayurvedic products, essential
oils, herbs, spices, supplements,
herbal remedies, incense, books
and other supplies. Must supply
resale certificate number or
practitioner license to obtain
catalog of more than 10,000
items.

Maharishi Ayur-Veda Products
International, Inc.
417 Bolton Road
P. O. Box 54
Lancaster, MA 01523
Ph: 800-ALL-VEDA
Fax: 508-368-7475

New Moon Extracts
P. O. Box 1947
Brattleborough, Vermont
05302-1947
Ph: 800-543-7279

Spectrum NaturalOmega 3 Oil
The Oil Company
133 Copeland Street
Petaluma, CA 94952

Universal Light, Inc.
P. O. Box 261
Dept. AN
Wilmot, WI 53192
Ph: 262-889 8571
Fax: 262-889 8591
E-mail:
universallight@lotuspress.com
Importer and Master Distribu-
tor for Vicco Herbal Toothpaste

Color, Sound, and Gems

PAZ
615 Carlisle S.E.
Albuquerque, NM 87106
Telephone: 505-268-6943
E-mail: ehecatl@wans.net
For open-backed gemstone set-
tings

Color Therapy Eyewear
C/O Terri Perrigone-Messer
P. O. Box 3114
Diamond Springs, CA 95619

Lumatron (light device)
C/O Ernie Baker
3739 Ashford-Dunwoody Rd.
Atlanta, GA 30139
Ph: 404-458-6509

Genesis (sound device)
Good Medicine
Attn: Tina Shinn
831 Grandview Ave.
Columbus, Ohio 43215
Ph: 614-488-5244

Essential Oil Supplies

Aromatherapy Supply
Unit W3
The Knoll Business Center
Old Shoreham Road
Hove, Sussex BN3 7GS
England

Aroma Vera
3384 South Robertson Pl.
Los Angeles, CA 90034
Ph: 800-669-9514

Auroma International
1100 Lotus Light Dr
Silver Lake, WI 53170 USA
Ph: 262-889-8569
Fax: 262- 889 8591
E-mail:
auroma@lotuspress.com
Website: www.auroma.net
Importer and master distributor of Auroshikha Incense, Chandrika Ayurvedic Soap and Herbal Vedic Ayurvedic products.

Earth Essentials Florida, Inc.
P. O. Box 35214
Sarasota, FL 34242
Ph: 800-370-3220
Fax: 941-346-0800
E-mail: earthess@aol.com
Rare Essential Oils

Fenmail Tisserand Oils
P. O. Box 48
Spalding, LINCS PE11 ADS
England

Internatural
P O Box 489
Twin Lakes, WI. 53181 USA
800-643 4221 (toll free order line)
262-889 8581 (office phone)
262-889 8591 (fax)
E-mail:
internatural@lotuspress.com
Website: www.internatural.com
Retail mail order and internet reseller of Ayurvedic products, essential oils, herbs, spices, supplements, herbal remedies, incense, books and other supplies.

Lotus Brands, Inc.
1100 Lotus Light Dr
Silver Lake, WI 53170 USA
Ph: 262-889-8561
Fax: 262-889-8591
E-mail:
lotusbrands@lotuspress.com
Website: www.lotuspress.com
Manufacturer and distributor of natural personal care and herbal products, massage oils, essential oils, incense and aromatherapy items.

Lotus Light Enterprises
1100 Lotus Drive
Silver Lake, WI 53170 USA
800-548 3824 (toll free order line)
262-889 8501 (office phone)
262-889 8591 (fax)
E-mail:
lotuslight@lotuspress.com
Website: www.lotuslight.com
Wholesale distributor of Ayurvedic products, essential oils, herbs, spices, supplements, herbal remedies, incense, books and other supplies. Must supply resale certificate number or practitioner license to obtain catalog of more than 10,000 items.

Private Universe
P. O. Box 3122
Winter Park, FL 32790
Ph: 407-644-7203

Oshadi Ayus -Quality Life Products
15, Monarch Bay Plaza, Ste. 346
Monarch Beach, CA 92629
Ph: 800-947-1008
Fax: 714-240-1104

Primavera
D 8961 Sulzberg
Germany
08376-808-0
(American Office)
110 Landing Court Unit B
Novato, CA 94945
Toll Free: 888-588-9830
Telephone: 415-209-6688
FAX: 415-209-6677

Original Swiss Aromatics
P. O. Box 606
San Rafael, CA 94915
Ph: 415-459-3998

Smitasha
26961 Ayamonte Dr.
Mission Viejo, CA 92692
Ph: 949-982-8777; 714-785-6891

Exercise Programs and Information

Diamond Way Ayurveda
P. O. Box 13753
San Luis Obispo, CA 93406
Ph/FAX: 805-543-9291
Toll Free: 877-964-1395
E-mail:
diamond.way.ayurveda@thegrid.net
(for Sotai, Tibetan Rejuvenation Exercises)

Natural Ingredients

Aloe Farms
P. O. Box 125
Los Fresnos, TX 78566
Ph: 800-262-6771
For aloe vera juice, gel, powder and capsules.

Arya Laya Skin Care Center
Rolling Hills Estates, CA 90274
For carrot oil.

Aubrey Organics
4419 North Manhattan Avenue
Tampa, FL 33614
For rosa mosquita oil and a large variety of natural cosmetics and shampoos.

Body Shop
45 Horsehill Road
Cedar Knolls, NJ 07927-2014
Ph: 800-541-2535
Aloe vera, nut and seed oils, cosmetics, make-up, brushes, loofahs, and much more.

Culpepper Ltd.
21 Bruton Street
London W1X 7DA
England
Variety of natural seed, nut, and kernal oils, essential oils, herbs, books, and cosmetics.

Desert Whale Jojoba Co.
P. O. Box 41594
Tucson, AZ 85717
Ph: 602-882-4195
For jojoba products and many other natural oils, including rice bran, pecan, macadamia nut and apricot kernal.

Everybody Ltd.
1738 Pearl Street
Boulder, CO 80302
Ph: 800-748-5675
Large variety of oils, oil blends, and cosmetics.

Flora Inc.
P. O. Box 950
805 East Badger Road
Lynden, WA 98264
Ph: 800-446-2110
For flax seed oil, herbal supplements for skin, hair, nails and cosmetics.

Green Earth Farm
P. O. Box 672
65 1/2 North 8th Street

Saguache, CO 81149
For calendula oil, creme, and herbal bath.

The Heritage Store, Inc.
P. O. Box 444
Virginia Beach, VA 23458
Ph: 804-428-0100
Castor oil, organic ghee, cocoa butter, massage oils, flowerwaters,
essential oils, cosmetics, and natural home remedies.

Internatural
P O Box 489
Twin Lakes, WI. 53181 USA
800-643 4221 (toll free order line)
262-889 8581 (office phone)
262-889 8591 (fax)
E-mail:
internatural@lotuspress.com
Website: www.internatural.com
Retail mail order and internet reseller of Ayurvedic products, essential oils, herbs, spices, supplements, herbal remedies, incense, books and other supplies.

Janca's Jojoba Oil and Seed Company
456 E. Juanita #7
Mesa, AZ 85204
Ph: 602-497-9494
Jojoba oil, butter, wax and seeds. Also a large variety of naturally
pressed unusual oils, such as camellia, kukui nut, and grapeseed. Also have clay, aloe products, essential oils, and their own line of cosmetics.

Lotus Brands, Inc.
1100 Lotus Light Dr
Silver Lake, WI 53170 USA
Ph: 262-889-8561
Fax: 262-889-8591
E-mail:
lotusbrands@lotuspress.com
Website: www.lotuspress.com
Manufacturer and distributor of natural personal care and herbal products, massage oils, essential oils, incense and aromatherapy items.

Lotus Light Enterprises
1100 Lotus Drive
Silver Lake, WI 53170 USA
800-548 3824 (toll free order line)
262-889 8501 (office ph.)
262-889 8591 (fax)
E-mail:
lotuslight@lotuspress.com
Website: www.lotuslight.com
Wholesale distributor of Ayurvedic products, essential oils, herbs, spices, supplements, herbal remedies, incense, books and other supplies. Must supply resale certificate number or practitioner license to obtain catalog of more than 10,000 items.

Weleda, Inc.
841 South Main Street
Spring Valley, NY 10977
For calendula oil and a large variety of natural cosmetics.

Pancha Karma Kitchen Equipment

Earth Fare
Attn: Roger Derrough
66 Westgate Parkway
Asheville, NC 28806
Ph: 704-253-7656
Carries hand grinders and suri-bachi clay pots and bowls.

Sesam Muhle Natural Products
RR1
Durham, Ontario
Canada, NOG 1RO
Ph: 519-369-6326
Carries a line of hand grinders and flakers for grains and legumes, made in Germany.

Taj Mahal Imports
1594 Woodcliff Drive, N.E.
Atlanta, GA 30329
Ph: 404-321-5940
Carries a full line of Indian kitchen equipment.

Pancha Karma Supplies

Vicki Stern
P. O. Box 1814
Laguna Beach, CA 92651
Ph: 949-494-8858
For steam boxes.

To Receive Pancha Karma

Ayurvedic Healings
Dr's Bryan & Light Miller
P. O. Box 35284
Sarasota, FL 34242
Ph: 941-346-3518
Fax: 941-346-0800
E-mail: earthess@aol.com

Website:
www.ayurvedichealing.com
Pancha Karma, Kaya Kalpa,
Jarpana, Shirodhara

Diamond Way Ayurveda
P.O. Box 13753
San Luis Obispo, CA 93406
Ph/FAX: 805-543-9291
Toll Free: 877-964-1395
E-mail:
diamond.way.ayurveda@thegrid.net

Dr. Lobsang Rapgay
2206 Benecia Ave.
Westwood, CA 90064
Ph: 310-282-9918

Spa Medicine

RejuveNation
Attn: Dr. Dennis Thompson
3260 47th St., #205A
Boulder, CO 80301
Ph: 303-417-0941
E-mail: drtdrt@concentric.net

Transformational Seminars

Vedic Astrology
American Council of Vedic
Astrology (ACVA)
P. O. Box 2149
Sedona, AZ 86339
Ph: 800-900-6595; 520-282-6595
Fax: 520-282-6097
Website: vedicastrology.org
E-mail: acva108@aol.com
Conferences, tutorial and train-
ing programs

American Institute of
Vedic Studies
Dr. David Frawley, Director
P. O. Box 8357
Santa Fe, NM 87504-8357
Ph: 505-983-9385
Fax: 505-982-5807
E-mail: vedicinst@aol.com
Website: www.vedanet.com
Correspondence courses in
Ayurveda and Vedic Astrology

Jeffrey Armstrong
4820 N. 35th St.
Phoenix, AZ 85018
Ph: 602-468-9448
Ayurvedic Astrologer, Author,
Lecturer, Teacher

Videos

Wishing Well Video
P. O. Box 1008
Dept. AN
Silver Lake, WI 53170
Ph: 262-889-8501
Wholesale & retail

Index

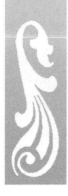

345

HERB AND MEDICINE INDEX

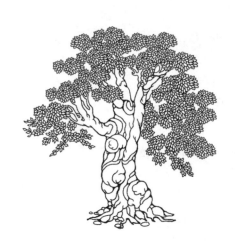

About the Authors

DR. DAVID FRAWLEY (Pandit Vamadeva Shastri) is one of the few Westerners recognized in India as a Vedic teacher (Vedacharya). His many fields of expertise include Ayurvedic medicine, Vedic Astrology, Yoga, 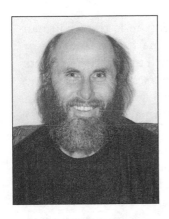 Vedanta and the Vedas themselves. He is the author of over twenty books on these subjects, including half a dozen books on Ayurveda. He has also written many articles for different newspapers, magazines and journals, and has taught and lectured throughout the world, including all over India.

Dr. Frawley is regarded as one of the 25 most influential Yoga teachers in America today according to the Yoga Journal. The Indian Express, one of India's largest English language newspapers, recently called him "a formidable scholar of Vedanta and easily the best known Western teacher of the Vedic wisdom." India Today, the Time Magazine of India, has called him, "Certainly America's most singular practicing Hindu." He also works closely with Dr. Deepak Chopra on various projects.

Currently Dr. Frawley is the director of the American Institute of Vedic Studies and the president of the American Council of Vedic Astrology (ACVA). He is on the editorial board for the magazine Yoga International. The American Institute of Vedic Studies features his extensive correspondence courses on Ayurveda and on Vedic Astrology.

PROF. SUBHASH RANADE is a leading academician and physician in the field of Ayurveda. He has written over 60 books on different subjects of 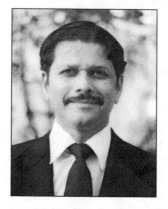 Ayurveda, which have been published in Marathi, Hindi, Malayalam, Polish, Japanese, Italian and German. He is the Executive Head and Professor of the Department of Ayurveda, Pune University and Executive Principle of Ashtang Ayurveda College in Pune, India.

At present he is the Chairman of the International Academy of Ayurveda in Pune which imparts Ayurveda courses, Panchakarma and Rejuvenative treatments for foreigners and Indians in Pune and Goa. He is also Chairman of the Ayurveda International Diffusing Association, Japan.

Professor Subhash Ranade has given many television interviews on Ayurveda, not only in India but in Poland, Italy and Germany as well. He has also attended many International and National seminars on Ayurveda and Yoga. He has written hundreds of articles on Ayurveda in various magazines, newspapers in India and abroad and is also on the editorial board of many Ayurvedic journals.

He has the honor of being visiting Professor to many Ayurvedic Institutes in the United States, the SEVA Academy in Munich, Germany, Ateneo Veda Vyasa, Savona, Italy and the Foundation for Health, Warsaw, Poland. His pioneering work in the field of CD-ROMS like Dhanvantari and Ayurvedic Massage and Marma Therapy have been whole-heartedly welcomed and highly appreciated by the Ayurvedic World.

Since 1981, he has visited and conducted hundreds of Ayurveda courses for medical practitioners in Europe, USA, Canada and Japan.